The Psychopharmacology Primer

A Guide to Understanding the Use of Psychotropic Medication for Individuals Who Have an Intellectual Disability and Mental Illness

Edward E. Hughes, M.A., LPA, NCP
Jerry McKee, Pharm.D., M.S., BCPP

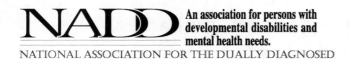

NATIONAL ASSOCIATION FOR THE DUALLY DIAGNOSED

132 Fair Street

Kingston, New York 12401

Library of Congress Number: 2007943417

ISBN: 1-57256-062-2

Printed in the United States of America

Contents

Preface

The *Primer* provides an overview of the use of psychotropic medication with individuals with intellectual disability. To the best of the authors' knowledge, this book summarizes the most up-to-date information available on this topic. Readers should understand, however, that the course of treatment for any particular individual will be based on factors unique to that individual. Because of this, there may be differences between the information in this book and what readers may observe with a family member or someone they support. Even so, this book should be of assistance to anyone who is advocating for effective treatment of mental health disorders through appropriate use of psychotropic medication.

Introduction

According to the World Health Organization, the definition of "health" is "a state of physical, mental, and social well-being and not merely the absence of disease or infirmity" (cited in Fletcher & Dosen, 1993). Thus, as Fletcher and Dosen note, mental health supports for individuals with intellectual disability should focus on stimulation of healthy mental development, prevention of psychiatric disorders, and effective treatment of psychiatric disorders. With regard to the last of these items, one of the most effective treatments for many mental health disorders is the prescription of psychotropic medication. For the sake of clarity, the term psychotropic medication, as used in this book, includes any drug prescribed to improve or stabilize someone's mood, behavior, or mental status.

The prescription of psychotropic medication for persons with intellectual disability has a controversial history. One of the most frequently voiced concerns has been that compared to other groups, far too many individuals with intellectual disability are given psychotropic medication. Early research (Lipman, 1970) supported this notion, noting that psychotropic medication rates approached 80% in some institutions. In addition,

Lipman found that almost 40% of those residing in institutions were taking major tranquilizers. Research conducted years later by Dimascio (1975) and by Tu and Smith (1979) found psychotropic medication rates of 42% and 53% percent, respectively.

In addition to relatively high rates of use, concerns have also been raised regarding the inappropriate use of psychotropic medications, primarily the antipsychotic agents, to sedate individuals with intellectual disability. In particular, it was feared that medication was being prescribed as a substitute for appropriate treatment or habilitation, for the convenience of staff, or that its use was simply not supported by a relevant diagnosis. Research conducted during the 1980's lent credence to at least some of these concerns, as Bates, Smeltzer, and Arnoczky (1986) found probable inappropriate use of psychotropics in 39% of the cases they reviewed. In addition, Heistad, Simmerman, and Doebler (1982) concluded that 44% of the individuals they reviewed had not benefited from their psychotropic drug treatment.

Some things have changed, however, since the 1970's and 1980's. More current research (Spreat, Conroy, & Fullerton, 2004) has reported that 35% of those receiving services from the Oklahoma intellectual disability service delivery system were treated with psychotropic medication. These researchers also found a threefold increase over ten years in the use of antidepressants as well as the more frequent prescription of anticonvulsant drugs to treat mental illness, both of which mirrored similar trends for individuals without intellectual disability during the same time period. The use of antipsychotic medication had not changed markedly, although there was a noticeable shift away from the older antipsychotics and towards the newer "atypical" medications.

Although these findings are limited in the extent to which they can be generalized to individuals in other places, they suggest that the rate of psychotropic medication usage has stabilized with individuals with intellectual disabilities. In addition, medication usage has also begun to reflect the prescribing patterns of the general population, albeit at a higher level. The question remains open, however, as to whether the medications prescribed are appropriate in terms of the underlying diagnosis or presenting symptoms. And it still appears to be the case that persons with intellectual disabilities are one of the most medicated groups in our society.

Chapter One

Guidelines for the Use of Psychotropic Medication

Despite the possible misuse of psychotropic medication in the past, it cannot be denied that these drugs may have a place in the treatment of mental illness, regardless of whether or not the person treated has an intellectual disability as well. The key is to ensure that the medications are being used appropriately. To this end, a set of guidelines has been published in *Psychotropic Medications and Developmental Disabilities: The International Consensus Handbook* (Reiss &: Aman, 1998). If followed, these guidelines should avoid needless risk and produce a good clinical outcome. Included are the following:

> ✓ Guideline: *Psychotropic medication shall not be used excessively, as punishment, for staff convenience, as a substitute for services, or in quantities that interfere with an individual's quality of life.*

This guideline should be understood to disallow not only excessively high dosages, but also the inappropriate long-term use of medication. In addition, this guideline means medication should not be used to control someone's behavior if that behavior is related to the appropriate expression of a personal right or is otherwise reasonable given the person's situation. It also captures the expectation that psychotropic medication is not intended to compensate for insufficient or poorly trained staff, inadequate environmental conditions or untreated medical issues, or to serve as a substitute for appropriate behavioral or educational interventions.

> ✓ Guideline: *Psychotropic medication must be used within a coordinated multidisciplinary care plan designed to improve the individual's quality oi life.*

The role of a multidisciplinary team in supporting individuals with intellectual disability, and in evaluating the appropriateness of psychotropic medications, has been shown to make a significant difference in the rates at which these medications are prescribed. Research conducted by LaMendola, Zaharia, and Carver (1980) and Schalock, Foley, Toulouse, and Stark (1985) found significant reductions of psychotropic medication when a multidisciplinary team was involved in the decision as to whether such medication should be employed.

> ✓ Guideline: *The use of psychotropic medication must be based on a psychiatric diagnosis or specific behavioral-pharmacological hypothesis resulting from a full diagnostic and functional assessment.*

In concrete terms, this guideline means that psychotropic medication should be prescribed only for a specific diagnosis included in the *Diagnostic and Statistical Manual of Mental Disorders: Fourth Edition -Text Revision* (*DSM IV-TR*) (American Psychological Association, 2000) or in response to a documented connection between the cause of unwanted behavior and the medication's known propensity to act on that cause. Thus psychotropic drugs should not be prescribed simply for "behaviors" or "aggression" without a proven cause-and-effect relationship.

> ✓ Guideline: *Written informed consent must be obtained from the individual, if competent, or the individual's guardian before the use of any psychotropic medication and must be periodically renewed.*

Embedded in this guideline is the principle that even if someone is not legally competent, he or she should be included to the extent possible in the decision to administer psychotropic medication. Informed consent by the person or an appropriate representative requires presentation of the risks and benefits of taking or not taking the medication, possible alternatives, and the right to refuse consent or revoke it at a later date. In addition, it is understood that all this information must be in a form that the individual can understand.

> ✓ Guideline: *Specific index behaviors and quality of life outcomes must be objectively defined, quantified, and tracked using recognized empirical measurement methods in order to monitor psychotropic medication efficacy.*

Index behaviors refer to observable signs or subjective feelings or sensations reported by the individual, by which changes in their condition may be measured. These signs, feelings, or sensations should be consistently monitored by reliable documentation systems or through the use of symptom-rating scales. Whatever documentation method is chosen, it should be implemented prior to the use of medication in order to establish a baseline for comparison with subsequent observations.

> ✓ Guideline: *The individual must be monitored for side-effects on a regular and systematic basis using an accepted methodology which includes a standardized assessment instrument.*

This guideline proposes that, in addition to any laboratory tests, scales or checklists designed to assess for side-effects should be used at least every 3 to 6 months, or as clinically indicated.

> ✓ Guideline: *If antipsychotic or other dopamine-blocking drugs are prescribed, the individual must be monitored for tardive dyskinesia on a regular and systematic basis using a standardized assessment instrument.*

Recognized instruments (e.g., AIMS, DISCUS) should be administered at least once every 6 months to assess for tardive dyskinesia. Even when a potential tardive dyskinesia-causing medication is discontinued, assessments should be repeated at one and two months afterwards to detect the possible emergence of withdrawal dyskinesia. In addition, if a person already has tardive dyskinesia but is no longer taking a dopamine-blocker, assessments should still be conducted at 6 to 12-month intervals.

> ✓ Guideline: *Psychotropic medication must be reviewed on a regular and systematic basis.*

It is recommended that at least every 3 months, or within 1 month after a medication or dosage change, the positive and negative effects of psychotropic medication should be formally reviewed. Those who should be a part of the review, either in person or by report, include the concerned individual and all relevant treatment team members including the psychiatrist or other knowledgeable clinician. One goal of these reviews should be to ensure that the lowest effective dosage and simplest possible drug regimen are utilized. And it is always important to ensure that therapeutic monitoring is in place (e.g., serum levels, CBC testing, renal functioning) for medications that require it.

In addition to the guiding principles noted above, the following actions can help to ensure the efficacy of an individual's medication regimen.

- ✓ Identify the changes expected as a result of taking of the medication.
- ✓ Identify the time frames by which these changes should occur.
- ✓ Develop a system to evaluate whether changes are occurring as planned (e.g., data tracking systems, rating scales).
- ✓ Identify one person to collect and summarize relevant data.
- ✓ Present data to the support team and psychiatrist on an ongoing basis.
- ✓ Regularly evaluate the accuracy of initial diagnostic impressions.
- ✓ Regularly evaluate the effectiveness of the medication regimen (i.e., positive and negative effects).
- ✓ Adjust diagnostic impressions and treatment approaches as indicated by data analysis.

Complementing the broad guidelines discussed above, the American Association on Mental Retardation has identified a number of specific practices that should be minimized (Rush & Frances, 2000). These include:

- ✓ Long term use of benzodiazepines (e.g., Ativan, Valium)
- ✓ Use of long-acting hypnotics (e.g., Dalmane, Doral)
- ✓ Long-term administration of anticholinergic medications (e.g., benzotropine)
- ✓ Use of anticholinergics in the absence of extrapyramidal side-effects
- ✓ High dosages of antipsychotic medications
- ✓ Employment of phenytoin, phenobarbital, or primidone as psychotropics or anticonvulsants

Medications on the so-called "Beers List" should be avoided whenever possible. The medications on this list, originally compiled by Dr. Mark Beers in 1991 and most recently updated in 2003, are outmoded or have replacement options which are much less likely to cause undesirable side-effects. Examples of medications on Beers List are Talwin, Darvon, Demerol, Sinequan, Elavil, Librium, Diabenese, Norpace, Ticlid, Bentyl, Equanil, and most muscle relaxants. Use of listed drugs may increase the potential for cognitive impairment, result in increased falls and fractures, or otherwise lead to a decrease in independent functioning.

Other Considerations

It may seem that the emphasis so far has been on low dosages of medication, administered for as short a time as possible. A more accurate sentiment, though, might be the right medication for the right length of time. One of the primary reasons for treatment failure with psychotropic medication, in fact, is failure to optimize the dosage or to allow adequate time for the medication to work. At the same time, another reason for poor therapeutic outcome is increasing a dose too rapidly. This practice often results in adverse side-effects, which then lead to medication discontinuation or poor adherence to the prescribed regimen. It is important to increase all medication dosages slowly and to decrease them slowly as well. With all that being said, it is still recommended to prescribe as few medications as possible and in the lowest effective dosages, thus reducing the risk of drug-to-drug interactions as well as adverse side-effects.

Another consideration, which may seem redundant, is that unnecessary or ineffective medications should always be discontinued. The logic of "If the problem is still occurring with the medications, imagine how bad it would be if they were stopped" is seriously flawed. The medications are not effective if the individual's problem persists.

Finally, it is wise to obtain all of a person's medication from the same pharmacy in order to facilitate screening for drug interactions. For example, serum levels of the drug Tegretol can be doubled when it is taken along with certain antibiotics (e.g., erythromycin). Such a problem can easily be prevented by medication interaction screening and preventive management by a pharmacist, but if both medications are not obtained from the same pharmacy, the problem may not be detected.

It can be seen, then, that a high degree of vigilance and even skepticism is required in the administration and management of psychotropic drugs. Through the responsible use of these medications, though, via the adherence to the guidelines and principles noted above, many persons with intellectual disability and mental illness will experience relief from their symptoms, improved adaptive functioning, greater independence, and a return to a fulfilling life.

Chapter Two

Dual Diagnosis – A Foundation of Understanding

Dual Diagnosis

The presence of mental illness in individuals with intellectual disability has been widely recognized by the scientific community for only about 30 years. Prior to this understanding, there was a commonly held belief that individuals with intellectual disability somehow enjoyed immunity from mental illness (Nezu, Nezu, & Gill-Weiss, 1992). The increased recognition and acceptance of mental health disorders in individuals with intellectual disability is due in part to the process of deinstitutionalization. Deinstitutionalization is the process by which individuals with intellectual disability moved from institutions into the community. This movement subsequently increased the visibility of individuals with a dual diagnosis and increased pressure on professionals to provide appropriate treatment.

Although psychiatric disorders are now accepted as occurring in individuals with intellectual disability, there continue to be barriers to the recognition and treatment of these disorders. Some of these barriers include: diagnostic overshadowing, behavioral overshadowing, medication masking, and episodic presentation. Below, these barriers are discussed in detail.

> **Diagnostic Overshadowing.** This term refers to overlooking or minimizing the signs of mental illness in an individual with intellectual disability (Reiss, Levitan, & Szysko, 1982). Mental illness may be overlooked or minimized because it is considered less debilitating than intellectual disability or because the symptoms of mental illness are attributed to the intellectual disability. As an example, difficulty concentrating may be attributed to intellectual disability when it is actually a symptom of depression.

> **Behavioral Overshadowing.** Behavioral Overshadowing refers to a tendency to identify psychopathology as learned behavior while failing to recognize it as an indicator of mental illness (Lowry, 1997). For example, a person's behavioral challenges may be thought to be related to "task avoidance" rather than a loss of motivation due to schizophrenia.

> **Medication Masking.** The sedative effects of certain medications (e.g., typical antipsychotic medications) can suppress, or mask, the presence of significant mental

health symptoms. For example, a person may be experiencing agitation related to depression but, due to limited communication skills, be unable to describe symptoms of their depression. If the person is prescribed a typical antipsychotic medication, the agitation may stop. However, the medication has not effectively treated the person's illness, and he or she may continue to suffer with symptoms of depression.

Episodic Presentation: Significant mental health symptoms may come and go in an unpredictable manner. If a person is not displaying symptoms when he or she is assessed by a mental health professional, the presence of a mental disorder may go undetected. As an example, an individual with bipolar disorder may be in a manic episode when an appointment is scheduled with his or her psychiatrist. By the time of the appointment, however, he or she may have cycled out of the manic episode and thus the symptoms of mania may no longer be present when examined by the psychiatrist.

Prevalence of Mental Health Disorders

Research compiled by Nezu, Nezu, & Gill-Weiss (1992) indicates the prevalence of mental illness in individuals with intellectual disability ranges from 5% to 100%. Reiss (1994) notes that some of the reasons for these widely varying prevalence rates include:

- ✓ Differing definitions of intellectual disability across studies
- ✓ Differing definitions of psychiatric disorders
- ✓ Differing methods for selecting subjects (e.g., institutions, random)
- ✓ Differing diagnostic approaches (e.g., chart review versus interviewing)

Despite the widely varying prevalence rates, existing studies confirm that individuals with intellectual disability are susceptible to the full range of mental health disorders. Experts generally agree that the most likely prevalence rate of mental illness among people with intellectual disability ranges from 20 to 35 percent (Nezu, Nezu, & Gill-Weiss, 1992). The *Diagnostic and Statistical Manual of Mental Disorders: Fourth Edition - Text Revision* (American Psychological Association, 2000), however, suggests that individuals with intellectual disability are three to four times more likely to experience mental health difficulties than individuals without intellectual disability. Although the exact prevalence of mental illness is unknown, it is generally accepted that individuals with intellectual disability are at increased risk for developing mental illness.

Proposed Causes for Increased Risk

Various reasons have been suggested for the relatively high prevalence rates of mental illness in individuals with intellectual disability. These factors are in addition to those generally accepted as causes for mental illness in the general population. Gualtieri (1988) reported two such widely accepted factors:

- ✓ Day-to-day life poses extraordinary challenges to individuals with intellectual disability and thus they experience increased stress.

- ✓ Individuals with intellectual disability have limited capacity to cope with stress and thus smaller stressors may be experienced as more intense.

The combination of increased stress or daily frustrations and a diminished ability to cope with stress is thought to contribute to the increased chance of mental illness. Gualtieri also notes that brain dysfunction and limited mental health care may also play a role.

Reiss (1994) and Ryan (1996) have proposed that various social and environmental factors experienced by individuals with intellectual disability may also help explain the prevalence of co-occurring mental illness. Proposed factors include:

- ✓ Rejection
- ✓ Segregation
- ✓ Lack of control over one's life
- ✓ Limited social support
- ✓ Limited vocational opportunities
- ✓ Poor self-image
- ✓ Limited social skills
- ✓ Labeling
- ✓ Increased rates of abuse and neglect

Psychiatric Diagnoses

Psychiatric diagnoses are useful insofar as they are accurate and help to direct needed treatment to improve a person's quality of life. A psychiatric diagnosis is made by looking for a collection of symptoms and then matching those symptoms to a specific disorder. The diagnostic standard for individuals with intellectual disability is the same as it is for anyone else. However, when considering a mental health diagnosis for an individual with intellectual disability, certain things should be kept in mind. Ryan (1996) proposes the following:

- Persons with intellectual disability are vulnerable to the full range of psychiatric conditions. In other words, people with intellectual disability can have the same disorders as people without intellectual disability.

- Since some medical problems and medication side-effects can look like mental health problems, these issues should be fully investigated prior to attempting to attribute symptoms or behavioral challenges to a psychiatric illness.

Many individuals with intellectual disability who are referred for a psychiatric evaluation present with challenging behaviors such as aggression, property destruction, and self-injury. It is important to remember, however, that while challenging behaviors may at times be related to the individual's mental illness, at other times they may not. Thus, behaviors that appear to be symptoms of a mental illness may simply be learned behaviors. Learned behaviors may be distinguished from behavior driven by psychiatric or medical illnesses, or simply better understood, by considering the following:

✓ If the symptom or behavior occurs in most or all settings it is more likely, but not necessarily, due to a psychiatric or medical condition.

✓ If the symptom or behavior is unresponsive to consistent behavioral interventions and habilitative programming, it is more likely related to a psychiatric or medical condition.

✓ If there are also changes in sleep, appetite, sexual, or daily functioning, the symptom or behavior is more likely to be attributable to a psychiatric or medical condition.

✓ If there are autonomic symptoms (e.g., tremors, high pulse rate, sweating), it is more likely the symptom or behavior is related to a psychiatric or medical condition.

✓ Individuals with intellectual disability frequently have limited means to express distress. Thus, the same behavior may mean something different every time it occurs. Therefore, the onset of a mental illness, or a medical problem, may worsen already existing challenging behaviors that are a result of faulty learning. When this occurs it is called baseline exaggeration.

✓ Individuals may display their usual challenging behavior that does not relate to a mental illness and simultaneously display other behavior that is indicative of a mental illness.

The manual that includes the criteria for all recognized mental health disorders is the *Diagnostic and Statistical Manual of Mental Disorders: Fourth Edition -Text Revision* (*DSM IV-TR*) (American Psychological Association, 2000). This manual uses a multi-axial system, which involves assessment on several different levels. The following table outlines this multi-axial system, providing a brief description of the definition and purpose of each axis.

DSM IV-TR Multi-axial System

Axis I	**Clinical disorders and mental illness**
Axis II	**Personality disorders and mental retardation**
Axis III	**Medical conditions relevant to understanding or managing the diagnosed mental disorder**
Axis IV	**Psychosocial or environmental problems affecting the diagnosis, treatment, or prognosis of the diagnosed mental disorder**
Axis V	**Clinician's rating of the individual's overall level of functioning (Global Assessment of Functioning - GAF)**

All relevant diagnoses should be listed for Axis I, II, and III. For example, a person may have two diagnoses on Axis II (e.g., mild mental retardation and borderline personality disorder). The use of the multi-axial system with an individual with dual diagnosis might look like this:

Axis I: **Schizoaffective Disorder, Bipolar Type**
Axis II: **Mild Mental Retardation**
Axis III: **Emphysema, Tardive Dyskinesia**
Axis IV: **Loss of job**
Axis V: **35 (range: 0-100)**

The process of obtaining the necessary information to diagnose a mental disorder typically starts with a clinical interview by a psychologist, psychiatrist, or other mental health professional. When such an interview is conducted, the following three factors must be kept in mind:

- Because of intellectual deficits, an individual with intellectual disability may have difficulty verbally reporting his or her thoughts or feelings.

Thus, there needs to be an increased focus on nonverbal communication. Preferably, the interview should occur in a natural setting or everyday context, such as a part of playing or participating in some activity.

- Individuals with intellectual disability who have language skills may have difficulty labeling their emotions or internal states. An example would be individuals who are reporting they are angry when they are really frightened.

- Concrete language and a lack of imagination by individuals with a dual diagnosis may lead clinicians to miss significant symptoms. An example would be an individual in a manic state who believes he can live on his own. While this claim might not sound like grandiosity, living on his own may be grossly out of proportion with the individual's skills and abilities and thus be consistent with grandiosity.

- It is important to remember that the usefulness of the clinical interview, regardless of the modifications made to the process, may decrease as verbal language and cognitive abilities decrease.

In light of some of the difficulties noted above, it is important that the clinical interview be supplemented by interviews with the individual's family, support staff, and other involved persons. Typically, these interviews seek to obtain information regarding the following:

- Recent Stressors: Since behavioral and psychiatric difficulties can result from changes in a person's life or environment, it is important to ensure that possible stressors are identified and then addressed as a part of treatment.

- Sleep Disturbance: Psychiatric disorders frequently disturb an individual's sleep. Information regarding changes in a person's sleep pattern may provide insights into the nature of the individual's disorder.

- Appetite Disturbance: Psychiatric disorders routinely result in appetite disturbances and associated weight loss or gain. Due to this, information related to appetite and weight is important to present to the assessing clinician.

- Activity Level: Some psychiatric disorders result in over-activity or under-activity and so it is important for any changes in activity level to be reported.

- Functioning Level: Many psychiatric disorders result in a decrease in an individual's ability to function independently. Specific examples of such declines should be presented to the clinician conducting the assessment.

- Family History of Mental Illness: An accurate family history helps in determining whether a particular disorder is likely to be present as a result of genetics or biological vulnerability.

In addition to providing the above information to the clinician conducting the interview, family members and support staff may also be called upon to assist in the completion of rating scales. Rating scales that can be used to assess for psychiatric and behavioral problems in individuals with intellectual disability include the ADD (Matson, 1997), PIMRA (Matson, 1988), DASH-II (Matson, 1995), and Reiss Screen (Reiss, 1988).

In addition to those previously reviewed, other activities should also be completed as a part of the diagnostic process. These include:

- ✓ Medical history and physical examinations
- ✓ A review of the person's psychiatric history via chart review or interview
- ✓ Direct observations in the person's natural environment
- ✓ Psychological testing
- ✓ Medication evaluations
- ✓ Functional behavioral assessment

Once all necessary information has been obtained, a diagnosis can be formulated. Even then, it is best to think of a diagnosis as tentative. Continued evaluation and assessment is needed to confirm the diagnosis.

Chapter Three

Clinical Disorders

Depression

Depression is a mental illness that affects the mind, body, and innermost feelings of an individual. While most people feel down from time to time, it is generally a natural and appropriate response to a particular life event. With depression, however, the symptoms are severe or long lasting. Depression may begin suddenly, possibly triggered by a personal loss or crisis, or the onset can be insidious. Depression can continue for months or years. It is possible for a person to have only one episode of depression, but it is more common for a person to experience multiple episodes during their lifetime. Depression affects millions of people each year but is often ignored or untreated. This is unfortunate as depression significantly disrupts work, family relations, and social life, yet it can usually be treated effectively.

Common symptoms of depression include:

- Sadness
- Irritability
- Loss of interest in daily life
- Hopelessness
- Loss of warm feelings for family or friends
- Low self-esteem
- Feelings of guilt or self-blame
- Negative thinking
- Inability to experience joy
- Feelings of emptiness
- Not tending to personal hygiene
- Physical complaints (e.g., headache, backache)
- Thoughts of death or suicide

Other common symptoms of depression, known as vegetative symptoms, include:

- Sleep disturbance
- Appetite disturbance
- Fatigue
- Impaired concentration
- Total loss of ability to experience pleasure
- Decreased interest in sex

Research conducted by Laman and Reiss (1987) found that depressed mood is among the most common psychiatric symptoms experienced by individuals with intellectual disability. In addition, Reiss and Rojahn (1993) found significantly higher rates of antisocial behavior, such as aggression or self-injury, for depressed individuals with intellectual disability versus non-depressed people with intellectual disability.

Because recognizing the symptoms of depression in individuals with intellectual disability may be difficult at times, various authors (Lowry, 1995; Ryan, 1996; Sovner & Lowrey, 1990) have devised the following list of behaviors, based on *DSM-IV-TR* criteria, that may be suggestive of the symptoms of depression.

DSM IV-TR SYMPTOM FOR DEPRESSION	PRESENTATION IN SOMEONE WITH INTELLECTUAL DISABILITY
Depressed Mood	<ul><li>Frequent unexplained crying</li><li>Decrease in laughter and smiling</li><li>General irritability and subsequent aggression or self-injury</li><li>Sad facial expression</li></ul>
Loss of Interest in Pleasure	<ul><li>No longer participates in favorite activities</li><li>Reinforcers no longer valued</li><li>Increased time spent in room alone</li><li>Refusals of most work/social activities</li></ul>
Weight Change/ Appetite Change	<ul><li>Measured weight changes</li><li>Increased refusals to come to table to eat</li><li>Unusually disruptive at meal times</li><li>Constant food seeking behaviors</li></ul>
Insomnia	<ul><li>Disruptive at bed time</li><li>Repeatedly gets up at night</li><li>Difficulty falling asleep</li><li>No longer gets up for work/activities</li><li>Early morning awakening</li></ul>
Hypersomnia	<ul><li>Over 12 hours of sleep per day</li><li>Naps frequently</li></ul>

DSM IV-TR SYMPTOM FOR DEPRESSION	PRESENTATION IN SOMEONE WITH INTELLECTUAL DISABILITY
Psychomotor Agitation	▪ Restlessness, fidgety, pacing ▪ Increased disruptive behavior
Psychomotor Retardation	▪ Sits for extended periods ▪ Moves slowly ▪ Takes longer than usual to complete activities
Fatigue/ Loss of Energy	▪ Needs frequent breaks to complete simple activity ▪ Slumped/tired body posture ▪ Does not complete tasks with multiple steps
Feelings of Worthlessness	▪ Statements like "I'm dumb," "I'm retarded," etc. ▪ Seeming to seek punishment ▪ Social isolation
Lack of Concentration/ Diminished Ability to Think	▪ Decreased work output in vocational setting ▪ Does not stay with tasks to completion ▪ Decrease in IQ upon retesting
Thoughts of Death	▪ Preoccupation with family members' deaths (e.g., increased interest in visiting grave, carrying photographs of deceased relatives, etc.) ▪ Talking about committing or attempting suicide ▪ Fascination with violent movies/television shows

Prior to diagnosing anyone with depression, it is important to first rule-out any possible medical causes for the individual's depressive symptoms. This is particularly true for individuals with intellectual disability as these individuals have an increased incidence of comorbid medical issues. When a medical illness is believed to be the cause for an individual's symptoms, the focus of treatment should be on treating the illness. Examples of illnesses that can cause symptoms consistent with depression are listed below.

Illnesses That May Cause Depression

- ✓ Anemia
- ✓ Hypothyroidism
- ✓ Cancer
- ✓ Chronic pain
- ✓ Chronic fatigue syndrome
- ✓ Congestive heart failure
- ✓ Diabetes
- ✓ Huntington's disease
- ✓ Cushing's disease
- ✓ Lyme's disease
- ✓ Multiple sclerosis
- ✓ Porphyria
- ✓ Sleep apnea
- ✓ Syphilis
- ✓ Wilson's disease

In addition to ensuring there are no medical illnesses that might be causing an individual's depression, it is also important to ensure the individual is not taking any medications or substances that might cause symptoms of depression as a side-effect. If such a medication or substance is found, the focus of treatment should be on modifying the person's medication regimen or discontinuing the substance use. Examples of medications and substances that can cause depression as a side-effect are listed below.

Substances That May Cause Depression

- ✓ Alcoholic drinks
- ✓ Anticonvulsants (e.g., phenytoin, carbamazepine)
- ✓ Antihypertensives (e.g., clonidine, propanalol)
- ✓ Antiparkinson medications (e.g., levodopa, amantadine)
- ✓ Barbituates (e.g., phenobarbital, secorbarbital)
- ✓ Benzodiazepines (e.g., diazepam, lorazepam)
- ✓ Calcium channel blockers (e.g., verapamil)

✓ Corticosteroids (e.g., prednisone)
✓ Hormonal medications (e.g., oral contraceptives)
✓ Pain medications (e.g., meperidine, codeine)

In addition to the above, withdrawal from alcohol and illegal drugs (e.g., cocaine, heroin, cannabis) can also result in depressive symptoms during the first three weeks after discontinuation of the substance.

Antidepressant Medications

Antidepressants work by restoring the balance of certain chemicals, called neurotransmitters, in the brain. Usually, antidepressants begin to bring relief from the symptoms of depression in four to six weeks. Some symptoms, such as fatigue or sleeping difficulties, may fade even earlier.

There are many kinds of antidepressants and the type prescribed will depend on each person's symptoms and other medical conditions. The four major groups of antidepressants include selective serotonin reuptake inhibitors (SSRIs), serotonin and norepinephrine reuptake inhibitors (SNRIs), Tricylics (TCAs), and Monoamine Oxidase inhibitors (MAOI). SSRIs (e.g., fluoxetine, paroxetine, sertraline, fluvoxamine, citalopram) and SNRIs (e.g., duloxetine, venlafaxine) generally cause fewer serious side-effects than other antidepressants. However, some individuals will not respond as well to SSRIs and SNRIs as they will to other antidepressants. Tricyclic antidepressants, such as amitriptyline, imipramine, and desipramine, are a bit older than SSRIs, but are still frequently used. Tricyclic antidepressants may be particularly effective when the person's depression has been severe, lasted a long time, or been associated with difficulty falling asleep at night.

MAOIs, such as phenelzine and tranylcypromine, are typically used when SSRIs, SNRIs, and Tricylic antidepressants have not been effective. The primary issue preventing more widespread use of MAOIs is that they can cause a potentially deadly hypertensive reaction when combined with certain tyramine containing foods (e.g., aged cheese, coffee, chocolate, red wine) or medications (e.g., certain pain killers or cold medications). Older MAOIs such as phenelzine and tranylcypromine inhibit both the A and B subtypes of MAO, thereby leading to the noted tyramine-related hypertensive problem. Selegiline, a newer MAOI, in lower doses is utilized to treat Parkinson's disease and when used via the transdermal patch works in such a way as to have no impact on MAO subtype A. Because of this, the transdermal delivery system of selegiline is less likely to cause serious adverse events. Even given this, a special diet is still recommended when using this medication.

Choosing a Treatment

Approximately two-thirds of individuals with depression can be treated successfully with medication alone. However, many individuals do not respond favorably to medication, have continued symptoms, frequently relapse, or simply prefer other treatment options. In these cases, treatment may consist of therapy, particularly cognitive-behavioral therapy, alone or in combination with medication. Of note is that it has been suggested that medication is always indicated when there are prominent and sustained vegetative symptoms.

Research on the efficacy of the use of antidepressants with individuals with intellectual disability and major depression has not generally met the rigorous scientific standards for clinical trials (e.g., double-blind placebo controlled). There are, however, numerous published reports, best described as case-studies (McGuire & Chicoine, 1996, Sovner, Foz, Lowry, & Lowry, 1993), that demonstrate antidepressant medications are effective in treating individuals with intellectual disability who have depressive disorders.

Course of Treatment

Antidepressants are usually started at a low dosage and then titrated up until the dose is in a therapeutic range. Subsequent to a relief in symptoms, antidepressants are typically continued for at least six months at the same dosage as the one that resulted in symptom improvement. Failure to continue the antidepressant for this period of time frequently results in a relapse of symptoms. If the individual has not had previous episodes of depression, the medication is then gradually reduced and ultimately discontinued. If the individual has had recurrent episodes of depression, generally three or more, the course of medication treatment may be life-long.

If an individual is experiencing major depression with psychotic features (e.g., delusions, hallucinations), antidepressants alone are usually ineffective. Generally, the most effective treatment is a combination of antidepressant and antipsychotic medication. For severe cases, or in instances where the person did not respond well to medication, electroconvulsive therapy (ECT) may be both necessary and helpful. In addition, ECT is also frequently used for treatment refractory or atypical depression. If ECT is ineffective for depression with psychotic features, the next step may include the use of a previously untried antidepressant or the use of a previously untried antidepressant in combination with lithium.

Side-effects and Precautions

Antidepressants, like any other medication, have side-effects. If the side-effects are intolerable, they can usually be managed by adjusting dosages or switching medications. Common potential side-effects for the different types of antidepressants are listed below.

Selective Serotonin Reuptake Inhibitors

- ✓ Difficulty sleeping
- ✓ Increase in anxiousness or restlessness
- ✓ Nausea
- ✓ Diarhea
- ✓ Headaches
- ✓ Reduced sexual interest or sexual dysfunction
- ✓ Potentially dangerous reaction when combine with MAOIs

Tricylic Antidepressants

- ✓ Dry mouth
- ✓ Constipation
- ✓ Difficulty urinating
- ✓ Light headedness
- ✓ Blurred visions
- ✓ Cardiac conduction problems

Monamine Oxidase Inhibitors

- ✓ Weight gain
- ✓ Dizziness
- ✓ Reduced sexual interest or sexual dysfunction
- ✓ Potentially deadly hypertensive reaction when combined with certain foods or medications (e.g., aged cheese, red wine, coffee, cold remedies, chocolate)

Serotonin and Norepinephrine Reuptake Inhibitors

- ✓ Nausea
- ✓ Sexual dysfunction
- ✓ Sweating
- ✓ Sleep disturbance
- ✓ Increased blood pressure

NOTE: In October, 2004, the FDA issued a directive to have product labeling for SSRI antidepressants contain a strong warning regarding a potential increased risk of suicide in adolescents treated with these medications. In an analysis of short-term (up to four months) trial data involving 24 trials and 4,400 patients, a 4% risk of suicidality was seen in the first four months, compared to a 2% placebo rate. No suicides occurred in these trials, which were not designed to evaluate suicidality as an endpoint. Similar findings have not occurred in adult trials with SSRI's. Consideration of the use of an antidepressant in a child or adolescent should balance the risk of potential increased suicidality with the clinical need. In addition, it is always sound clinical practice to closely observe any individual undergoing a medication trial for worsening symptoms and to communicate with the clinical service provider. Unfortunately, since this warning was issued, the suicide rate among U.S. residents less than age 20 increased by 18% (from 2003 to 2004), perhaps related to declining rates of antidepressant use due to the hearings leading up to the warning being issued.

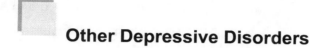

Other Depressive Disorders

Dysthymic Disorder

Dysthymic disorder is a depressive disorder that is characterized by mild depressive symptoms that are present for at least two years. Individuals with this disorder are able to function fairly well on a day-to-day basis, but their relationships and career eventually begin to suffer as a result of their symptoms. In addition, it is not uncommon for individuals with dysthymic disorder to also experience episodes of major depression as well. When this occurs, it is often referred to as "double depression." Symptoms of dysthymic disorder include:

- Fatigue
- Low self-esteem
- Irritability
- Diminished interest in life or enjoyment
- Low energy
- Negative thinking
- Sleep difficulties

In multiple studies, antidepressant medication has been shown to be effective in treating dysthymia. Prozac and Tofranil have been shown to be particularly effective. The response rate for the treatment of dysthymia with antidepressant medication is around sixty-two percent. In addition, the use of psychotherapy, particularly cognitive-behavioral therapy, can be an effective treatment for some individuals with dysthymia.

Premenstural Dysphoric Disorder

Premenstrual Dysphoric Disorder (PMDD) is a condition characterized by severe emotional and physical problems that are linked to a woman's menstrual cycle. Symptoms typically begin in the second half of a woman's cycle and end as menstruation begins or shortly thereafter. PMDD is often conceptualized as a much more severe form of PMS and affects about five-percent of women. PMDD is very disruptive to women's lives and is characterized by:

- Anxiety
- Tension
- Irritability
- Mood lability
- Depression

Although no single medication has proven itself to be consistently better than others, SSRIs are the preferred treatment. While all the drugs in this class may be helpful, only fluoxetine, paroxetine controlled-release, and sertraline have been approved by the FDA to treat PMDD. There continues to be some debate as to whether it is best to treat PMDD continuously, or with PRN dosing. Fluoxetine, paroxetine controlled-release, and sertraline, however, are approved for both continuous and intermittent use. While most of the research on the treatment of PMDD has not included individuals with intellectual disability, case studies have been published (Mavromatis, 1999) supporting the use of SSRIs for individuals with intellectual disability and PMDD.

Generally, SSRIs provide relief from the symptoms of PMDD during the first month of treatment. However, if adjustments in dosages are necessary, it may take two or three menstrual cycles to get a full response. It is also noted that, in addition to medication, psychobehavioral interventions (e.g., coping skills training, relaxation training) and nutritional interventions (e.g., vitamin, minerals, dietary modifications) may have a positive impact on the symptoms of PMDD.

Seasonal Affective Disorder

Seasonal Affective Disorder (SAD) is a type of depression that follows the seasons, with the most common type being winter associated depression. Winter SAD typically begins in the late fall or early winter and subsides by summer. A much more rare form of SAD, known as summer depression, begins in late spring or early summer and ends by winter. Symptoms of SAD keep coming back year after year and tend to come and go at about the same time each year. Some of the more common symptoms of SAD include:

- Change in appetite (e.g., craving sweet or starchy foods)
- Decreased energy
- Fatigue
- Increased desire for sleep
- Irritability
- Social avoidance
- Increase in emotional sensitivity
- Difficulty concentrating
- Somatic complaints (e.g., headaches)
- Loss of interest in life

Treatment for SAD may include the use of antidepressant medication, particularly the SSRIs. Often, however, the preferred treatment for SAD is the use of light therapy via specially made light boxes or visors. These devices are used during the time of year the individual is likely to experience SAD, with the individual using them for about 30 minutes a day. Although there are no controlled studies evaluating the efficacy of light therapy for individuals with intellectual disability and SAD, research (Altabet, Newman, and Watson-Johnson, 2002) suggests light therapy can reduce depressive symptoms in individuals with intellectual disability.

Bipolar Disorder

Bipolar disorder is an illness that causes extreme mood swings. A person with bipolar disorder may have periods of mania, depression, and normal moods. During an episode of mania, an individual will typically have an oversupply of confidence and energy that may lead to reckless or dangerous behavior as well as impaired judgment. The length of a manic or depressed cycle may last from days to months. Without treatment, bipolar disorder can lead to poor job performance, financial difficulties, problems with family and friends, and death from reckless behavior or suicide.

There are two primary types of bipolar disorder. The first type, bipolar I, is characterized by one or more manic or mixed episodes. A mixed episode is when manic and depressed symptoms occur simultaneously. For example, a person may be experiencing pressured speech and psychomotor agitation at the same time they feel hopeless and worthless. Often, individuals with bipolar I have also had one or more major depressive episodes.

Bipolar II is characterized by one or more major depressive episodes and at least one hypomanic episode. A hypomanic episode is a less intense episode of mania. The individual experiences an increased level of energy, moves at a more rapid pace, and generally feels, and may appear, more productive. By its less intense nature, compared to that of a manic episode, a hypomanic episode may go undetected. Because manic episodes are more easily observed than hypomanic episodes, we will review the symptoms of mania.

Symptoms of bipolar I disorder vary from one person to another, but during a manic episode symptoms may include:

- Feeling invincible or overconfident
- Extreme activity
- Sleeping less without feeling tired
- Irritability
- Racing thoughts
- Rapid speech

- Sexual promiscuity or sexually inappropriate behavior
- Talking in a loud and fast manner
- Being easily distracted
- Poor judgement
- Delusions about having special abilities

Many of the symptoms associated with a manic episode are often associated with intellectual disability (e.g., poor judgment, distractibility, excessive activity). Thus, the key in determining if an individual with intellectual disability is experiencing a manic episode is to compare the person's current functioning with their previous functioning. Because recognizing the symptoms of mania may be difficult at times, the following is a list of behaviors that may be observed and are suggestive of the symptoms of mania in persons with an intellectual disability (Sovner & Lowery, 1990; Ryan, 1996; Lowry, 1995).

DSM IV-TR SYMPTOMS OF MANIA	PRESENTATION IN SOMEONE WITH INTELLECTUAL DISABILITY
Euphoric, Elevated or Irritable Mood	<ul><li>Smiling, hugging or being affectionate with people who previously were not favored by the individual</li><li>Aggression towards previously favored person</li><li>Boisterousness</li><li>Over-reactivity to small incidents</li><li>Extreme excitement</li><li>Excessive laughing and giggling</li><li>Self-injury associated with irritability</li><li>Enthusiastic greeting of everyone</li></ul>
Decreased Need for Sleep	<ul><li>Behavioral challenges when prompted to go to bed</li><li>Constantly getting up at night</li><li>Seems rested after not sleeping (i.e., not irritable due to lack of sleep as is common in depression)</li><li>Works on activities in room during the night</li></ul>
Inflated Self-esteem/ Gradiosity	<ul><li>Making improbable claims (e.g., is a staff member, has mastered all necessary skills, etc.)</li><li>Wearing excessive make-up</li><li>Dressing provocatively</li><li>Demanding rewards</li></ul>
Flight of Ideas	<ul><li>Disorganized speech</li><li>Thoughts not connected</li><li>Quickly changing subjects</li></ul>

DSM IV-TR SYMPTOMS OF MANIA	PRESENTATION IN SOMEONE WITH INTELLECTUAL DISABILITY
More Talkative/ Pressure Speech	<ul><li>Increased singing</li><li>Increased swearing</li><li>Perseverative speech</li><li>Screaming</li><li>Intruding in order to say something</li><li>Non-verbal communication increases</li><li>Increase in vocalizations</li></ul>
Distractibility	<ul><li>Decrease in work/task performance</li><li>Leaving tasks uncompleted</li><li>Inability to sit through activities (e.g., favorite tv show)</li></ul>
Agitation/Increase in Goal Directed Behavior	<ul><li>Pacing</li><li>Negativism</li><li>Working on many activities at once</li><li>Fidgeting</li><li>Aggression</li><li>Rarely sits</li></ul>
Excessive Pleasurable Activities	<ul><li>Increase in masturbation</li><li>Sexualizing previously platonic relationships</li><li>Teasing others</li><li>Giving away/spending money</li></ul>

Prior to diagnosing anyone with bipolar disorder, it is important to first rule-out possible medical causes for the individual's symptoms. When a medical illness is believed to be the cause for an individual's symptoms, the focus of treatment should be on treating the illness.

Ilnesses That May Cause Mania

- ✓ Delirium
- ✓ Multiple sclerosis
- ✓ Encephalitis
- ✓ Influenza
- ✓ Brain tumors
- ✓ Hyperthyroidism

In addition to ensuring there are no medical illnesses that might be causing an individual's mania, it is also important to ensure the individual is not taking any medications or substances that might cause symptoms of mania as a side-effect. If such a medication or substance is found, the focus of treatment should be on modifying the person's medication regimen or discontinuing the substance use. Examples of medications and substances that can cause symptoms of mania as a side-effect are listed below.

Substances That May Cause Mania

- ✓ Amphetamines
- ✓ Antidepessants
- ✓ Bromides
- ✓ Cannabis
- ✓ Cocaine
- ✓ Steroids
- ✓ Stimulants

Mood Stabilizers

Mood stabilizers are medications used in the treatment of disorders characterized by rapid and unstable mood shifts such as bipolar disorder and borderline personality disorder. Many of the mood stabilizers were originally developed to treat seizure disorders. Anticonvulsants used as mood stabilizers include divalproex, carbamazepine, lamotrigine, oxcarbazepine, topiramate, and gabapentin. Lithium, which is not an anticonvulsant, is one of the oldest mood stabilizers and remains a first-line treatment for disorders such as bipolar. In addition, lithium is effective in treating the depression associated with bipolar disorder. Atypical antipsychotic medications (e.g., zyprexa) are also used as mood stabilizers. However, not all atypical antipsychotic medications have indications for mood stabilization and, even when they do, they are not generally considered as a first-line treatment. In addition, it has been conjectured that omega-3 fatty acid may have a mood stabilizing effect when used with mood stabilizers. Well designed rigorous research to verify this, however, has yet to be published.

Mood stabilizers are effective in treating mania and preventing shifts between depression and mania. With the exception of lamotrigine, however, mood stabilizers are generally less effective in treating depression. Often, an antidepressant is prescribed in addition to a mood stabilizer to treat depression. This, however, brings some risks as antidepressants can induce mania or psychosis in individuals with bipolar disorder, especially when the person is not already taking a mood stabilizer.

Choosing a Treatment

Typically, if an individual is presenting with symptoms of mania, the recommended approach is to begin treatment with a mood stabilizer. If the individual is presenting with psychotic symptoms or significant agitation, and since individuals may not show a response to the medication for ten to fourteen days, the mood stabilizer may be augmented with an antipsychotic medication or a benzodiazepine. Once the individual has stabilized, these medications are typically tapered away. If the individual is presenting with symptoms of depression, the general treatment approach is to start with a mood stabilizer. If the mood stabilizer is not effective in remedying the symptoms, an antidepressant medication may then be added. Treatment with mood stabilizing medication is life-long as evidence suggests that failure to continue taking medication results in relapse. In addition, experts in the field (Suppes & Dennehy, 2005) have suggested that in a majority of cases, two or more medications are typically needed for effective treatment. In addition to medication, treatment for bipolar disorder often also includes psychoeducational, problem solving/coping skill, and interpersonal interventions.

While most of the research on the treatment of bipolar disorder has involved individuals without intellectual disability, there are a collection of studies, ranging from adequately designed controlled trials to case presentations, that support the use of lithium, anticonvulsants, and atypical antipsychotics for the treatment of bipolar disorder in individuals with intellectual disability (Pary, Friedlander, & Capone, 1999; Burgess, 2002).

Side-effects and Precautions

Mood stabilizers, like any other class of medication, have side-effects. If the side-effects are intolerable, they can usually be managed by adjusting dosages or switching medications. Common potential side-effects for the different types of mood stabilizers are listed below.

Lithium

- ✓ Nausea
- ✓ Diarrhea
- ✓ Vomiting
- ✓ Hand tremor
- ✓ Polyuria (excessive urination)
- ✓ Polydispsia (excessive thirst)
- ✓ Edema
- ✓ Dry mouth

Side-effects of chronic, or long term, lithium use include:

- ✓ Hyopothyroidism
- ✓ Kidney damage

Signs of lithium toxicity include:

- ✓ Lethargy
- ✓ Slurred speech
- ✓ Ringing in the ears

- ✓ Vomiting
- ✓ Tremor
- ✓ Seizures
- ✓ Delirium
- ✓ Ataxia
- ✓ Cardiac conduction abnormalities

Anticonvulsant Mood Stabilizers

- ✓ Nausea
- ✓ Sedation
- ✓ Weight Gain
- ✓ Rashes
- ✓ Hand tremor
- ✓ Blood dyscrasias
- ✓ Ataxia

Atypical Antipsychotics

- ✓ Dry mouth
- ✓ Constipation
- ✓ Blurred vision
- ✓ Drowsiness
- ✓ Obesity
- ✓ Diabetes
- ✓ High cholesterol

Obsessive Compulsive Disorder

Obsessive compulsive disorder (OCD) is characterized by obsessive thoughts or images and, at times, compulsions. Obsessive thoughts or images are recurrent and interfere with daily life and lead to anxiety and discomfort. In addition, the person experiencing the obsessions would like them to stop and, at least initially, understands them to be irrational. Compulsions are repeated behaviors or activities that are performed in response to the obsessive thoughts or images. The individual typically derives no pleasure from the compulsive behavior. They may, however, experience a decrease in the anxiety created by the obsessive thought or image by yielding to the compulsion. OCD in the general population is associated with above average intelligence and thus it would be expected to occur at relatively low rates in individuals with intellectual disability. However, research cited by Lew (1995) found that people with intellectual disability are diagnosed with OCD at rates higher than the general population.

Because of poor or limited communication and a lack of insight on the part of some individuals with intellectual disability, it may be quite difficult to distinguish between a compulsion and the repetitive or stereotypic behavior often seen in persons with intellectual disability. Typically, individuals engaging in stereotypical or repetitive behavior do not seem to resist the behavior or to be distressed by it. In contrast, compulsive behaviors may be resisted by the individual. Further, attempts to interrupt compulsions are more likely to result in aggression or other behavioral challenges (Vitiello, Spreat, & Behar, 1989).

Symptoms of OCD vary from one person to another, but may include:

- Spending hours washing hands and other body parts
- Cleaning objects repeatedly for fear of germs
- Repeatedly checking things like whether the stove is turned off
- Repeating certain actions such as dressing or grooming activities
- Hoarding objects others would throw away
- Spending hours organizing a desk or room
- Ruminating on thoughts, prayers, sequences of numbers, etc.

Gedye (1992) has created the Compulsive Behavior Checklist which is designed specifically for people with intellectual disability. The checklist is broken down into five categories of compulsions as outlined in the following table.

Compulsive Behavior Checklist

Checklist	Type of Compulsion	Example
•	Ordering Compulsions	Arranging objects into a certain order or in a certain area
•	Completeness/Incompleteness	Closing doors or dressing and undressing oneself
•	Cleaning/Tidiness Compulsions	Repeatedly cleaning one certain body part
•	Checking/Touching Compulsions	Touching items repeatedly
•	Grooming Compulsions	Checking self in mirror excessively

It is important to remember that this checklist cannot confirm a diagnosis of OCD, but can be helpful in collecting information when a diagnosis of OCD is being considered.

Treatment

The treatment of choice for OCD includes the use of Selective Serotonin Reuptake Inhibitors (SSRIs) or clomipramine (TCA), usually in combination with behavior therapy. In the absence of behavior therapy, relapse is likely upon discontinuation of medication and thus medication use is generally life-long. Subsequent to the initiation of SSRIs, individuals may experience a gradual improvement in symptoms for up to twelve months. After about a year, improvement usually stabilizes. Generally, treatment is not curative but does result in an improvement of symptoms and an increased quality of life.

The primary research with regards to the treatment of OCD has been with individuals without intellectual disability. However, case studies supporting the use of SSRIs and clomiprimine in individuals with intellectual disability and OCD are present in the literature (Cook, Terry, Heller, & Leventhal 1990; Bodfish and Madison, 1993). If SSRI or clomipramine therapy fails, augmentation strategies have been proposed with medications such as buspirone. However, significant evidence of improvement with such trials is lacking. Atypical antipsychotic agents have shown encouraging results when used in augmentation trials for OCD, with risperidone currently having the most supportive evidence when used at low dosages (0.5-2 mg per day).

Posttraumatic Stress Disorder

Posttraumatic stress disorder (PTSD) is an emotional and psychological reaction that occurs in individuals who have experienced or witnessed a traumatic event. After the trauma, individuals may feel their lives have changed and what was once seen as a safe world is suddenly seen as dangerous and unpredictable. Symptoms of PTSD last for more than a month and may lead to problems at work as well as conflicts with friends and family.

Research cited by Reiss (1994) indicates there is preliminary evidence to suggest that individuals with lower levels of intelligence and education are more susceptible to developing PTSD in response to a traumatic event. Further, research conducted by Sobsey and Varnhagen (1991) indicates individuals with intellectual disability are more likely to encounter physical or sexual abuse during their lifetime than are individuals without intellectual disability. Thus, individuals with intellectual disability would be expected to be quite vulnerable to PTSD.

Traumatic events can occur to anyone and include such things as:

- ✓ Abuse
- ✓ Violent crime
- ✓ Rape or sexual assault
- ✓ Natural disasters
- ✓ Fires
- ✓ Car accidents
- ✓ Unexpected death of a loved one

Symptoms of PTSD vary from one person to another, but may include:

- Recurring memories or flashbacks
- Nightmares
- Physical problems like headaches, nausea, and chest pain
- Feelings of sadness, hopelessness, or loneliness
- Lack of interest in pleasurable activities
- Guilt over surviving the traumatic event
- Insomnia
- Difficulty concentrating
- Irritability or angry outbursts

In children, the symptoms of PTSD may include:

- Reliving the event through play
- Tantrums
- Difficulty separating from parents
- Thumb sucking or bed wetting

Professionals in the field of dual diagnosis (Charlot, 1997) have suggested that it may be appropriate, based on a developmental approach, to use the diagnostic criteria for children when considering the presence of a mental health disorder in an individual with intellectual disability. Thus, the criteria related to a child's experience of PTSD may provide more useful diagnostic information than the criteria intended for adults.

Treatment

Although psychotherapy is effective for the treatment of PTSD, regardless of whether the person has an intellectual disability, psychotropic medications may be helpful in reducing some symptoms of PTSD. For example, transient psychotic symptoms may be responsive to a short-term course of antipsychotic medication. Intrusive symptoms like nightmares, flashbacks, and anxiousness may be treated with SSRIs. Emerging research also suggests the use of clonidine or beta blockers (e.g., propanolol), when given shortly after a traumatic event, may help to prevent progression to the more chronic forms of PTSD.

Schizophrenia

Schizophrenia is a mental illness that affects the way a person thinks, feels, and acts. Individuals with schizophrenia may have trouble concentrating or organizing their thoughts. This may appear in speech that contains many unrelated thoughts or simply a collection of words or sounds. Emotions may come out inappropriately such as crying at jokes, or laughing at something considered sad or disturbing. Or, the person may become unable to express feelings at all. The person may also have a diminished ability to start or complete activities.

While some debate on the issue remains, authorities suggest that schizophrenia can be diagnosed in individuals with intellectual disability regardless of the degree of cognitive impairment (Ryan, 1996). The ability to definitively diagnose schizophrenia in individuals with intellectual disability, however, is inversely correlated to the degree of cognitive impairment. In addition, caution must be exercised when diagnosing individuals with intellectual disability with schizophrenia, as developmentally appropriate self-talk, imaginary friends, fantasy play, and beliefs based on faulty learning may be confused with hallucinations and delusions (Hurley, 1999). Further, caution is also indicated because delusions and hallucinations are not specific to schizophrenia, but can be present during the course of other psychiatric disorders, such as depression and bipolar disorder.

Without treatment, individuals with schizophrenia may have difficulty keeping a job, maintaining relationships with others, and taking care of themselves. Most individuals with schizophrenia will have periodic worsening and improvement of their symptoms. However, with the proper medical and social support many people with schizophrenia can lead fulfilling and productive lives.

Symptoms of schizophrenia vary from person to person and often come and go in cycles. Symptoms include:

- Firmly held false beliefs called delusions. For example, a person may believe that he or she is famous, or that other people are trying to hurt them.
- Hearing, seeing, smelling, tasting, or feeling things that are not there. These types of experiences are called hallucinations.
- Shifting from one thought to another with no obvious connection, making up words, or using sounds or rhymes in place of words.
- Engaging in behaviors that do not seem to have a purpose.
- Avolition (a lack of interest in, or motivation to complete, activities)
- Anhedonia (an inability to experience pleasure)

Other symptoms of schizophrenia include:

- Making odd or repetitive movements.
- Dressing inappropriately for the weather
- Not moving for hours or pacing constantly
- Ignoring personal hygiene
- Avoiding social contact
- Flat or blunted affect
- Decrease in amount of speech

Because recognizing the symptoms of schizophrenia may be difficult, Myers and Peuschel (1996) and Ryan (1996) have compiled a list of behavioral equivalents which may be demonstrated by individuals with intellectual disability that are suggestive of the symptoms of schizophrenia. The following table outlines this list.

DSM IV-TR SYMPTOM FOR SCHIZOPHRENIA	PRESENTATION IN INDIVIDUAL WITH INTELLECTUAL DISABILITY
Delusion	<ul><li>New avoidance or fear behaviors</li><li>Irrational beliefs not previously expressed</li><li>Bizarre accusations regarding others</li><li>Sudden refusal to take medications (i.e., belief medication is poison)</li><li>Carefully inspecting food as if it has been poisoned</li></ul>
Hallucination	<ul><li>Talking to non-existent people</li><li>Turning head as if listening to sounds no one else hears</li><li>Reporting on conversations not heard by others</li><li>Sniffing air as if smelling something not smelled by others</li><li>Pushing unseen objects off of body</li><li>Covering eyes or ears as if to block out hallucinations</li><li>Sudden appearance of "shadow boxing"</li></ul>
Disorganized Speech	<ul><li>Regression in language skills</li><li>Decrease in amount of language</li><li>Speech no longer makes sense</li></ul>
Grossly Disorganized/ Catatonic Behavior	<ul><li>Sudden appearance of new unusual mannerisms</li><li>Assuming the same position for long periods of time</li><li>Regression in performance of previously acquired skills</li></ul>
Negative Symptoms	<ul><li>Lack of expression of emotions (must represent a change from baseline)</li><li>Lack of interest in previously enjoyed activities</li><li>Reinforcers no longer effective</li><li>Speech no longer present</li></ul>

Prior to diagnosing anyone with schizophrenia, it is important to first rule-out any possible medical causes for the individual's symptoms. When a medical illness is believed to be the cause for an individual's symptoms, the focus of treatment should be on treating the illness. Examples of illnesses that can cause psychotic symptoms are listed below.

Illnesses That May Cause Psychosis

- ✓ Addison's disease
- ✓ Cushing's disease
- ✓ Delirium
- ✓ Dementia
- ✓ Huntington's chorea
- ✓ Hypothyroidism
- ✓ Hyperthyroidism
- ✓ Lupus
- ✓ Multiple sclerosis
- ✓ Porphyria

In addition to ensuring there are no medical illnesses that might be causing an individual's psychotic symptoms, it is also important to ensure the individual is not taking any medications or substances that might cause these symptoms as a side-effect. If such a medication or substance is found, the focus of treatment should be on modifying the person's medication regimen or discontinuing the substance use. Examples of medications and substances that can cause psychotic symptoms as a side-effect are listed below.

Substances That May Cause Psychosis

- ✓ Antiinflamatory drugs (e.g., steroids)
- ✓ Anticholinergic drugs
- ✓ Illegal drugs (e.g., cocaine, amphetamines, LSD)

In addition to the above, withdrawal from alcohol and drugs (e.g., barbituates, benzodiazepines) can also result in psychotic symptoms.

Antipsychotic Medications

Antipsychotic medications are primarily used to treat schizophrenia and other psychotic disorders. However, some antipsychotic medications have proven useful in the treatment of mood disorders, such as bipolar disorder and depression. Antipsychotic medications help restore the balance of chemicals in the brain and this results in the improvement of a person's symptoms. There are two kinds of antipsychotic medication, and they work in different ways. The first type, referred to as first generation or typical antipsychotic medications, primarily affect the levels of dopamine in certain areas of the brain. Examples of traditional antipsychotic medications include haloperidol, chlorpromazine, thioridazine, and thiothixene.

The second type of antipsychotic medications are the atypical, or second generation, antipsychotics. These medications affect other chemicals in the brain in addition to dopamine. Examples of atypical antipsychotic medications include risperidone, quetiapine, olanzapine, ziprasidone, and clozapine. Atypical antipsychotics are often used instead of traditional antipsychotic medications. The potential benefits of ayptical antipsychotics are two fold. First, they have been shown to help individuals who showed no improvement with typical antipsychotic medication, and, second, they generally have fewer intolerable extrapyramidal side-effects compared to older agents (e.g., typical antipsychotics).

Choosing a Treatment

Both typical and atypical antipsychotic medications are effective in treating the positive symptoms of schizophrenia (e.g., delusions, hallucinations, disorganization). Atypical antipsychotics, however, have shown superior efficacy compared to typical antipsychotics in treating the negative symptoms (e.g., avolition, anhedonia) of schizophrenia. In general, the choice of antipsychotic medication is driven primarily by consideration of the side-effect profile of the different medications. An exception, is that the more sedating antipsychotics may be indicated if the individual is also significantly agitated.

Research on the efficacy of the use of antipsychotics with individuals with intellectual disability and schizophrenia has not met the standards for clinical trials (e.g., double-blind placebo controlled). There are, however, published reports (Boulding et al., 2005), best described as open-label case-studies, that antipsychotic medications are effective in treating individuals with intellectual disability who have schizophrenia. Moreover, the AAMR Consensus Guidelines (Rush & Frances, 2000) recommend the use of atypical antipsychotics for individuals with schizophrenia and intellectual disability.

Course of Treatment

Antipsychotic medications are usually started at a relatively low dose and then titrated upward until there is a clinically significant reduction in symptoms. Emotional dyscontrol and agitation are usually the first symptoms to improve. Over time, improvement is then seen in hallucinations, delusions, and disordered thinking. If it is the person's first episode, the usual course is to find the lowest effective dose and continue to treat for about twelve months. If a person has had multiple episodes, the usual course is to find the lowest effective dose and continue treatment long-term. In addition, psychosocial treatments often serve as a useful adjunct to psychotropic medication. Typically, these involve:

- ✓ Education about the signs and symptoms of schizophrenia.
- ✓ Developing plans of action for the person to implement when symptoms re-emerge.
- ✓ Developing strategies to help the person cope with symptoms.
- ✓ Developing strategies for improving social skills and/or activities of daily living.
- ✓ Individual and group therapy to deal with the emotional and practical challenges of schizophrenia
- ✓ Social skills training
- ✓ Recreation therapy
- ✓ Vocational training

Side-effects and Precautions

Antipsychotics, like any other medication, have side-effects. If the side-effects are intolerable, they can usually be managed by adjusting dosages or switching medications. Side effects are highly variable, even within the same class of medication. Some common potential side-effects of antipsychotic medications include:

Typical/First Generation Anitpsychotic Medications

- ✓ Extrapyramidal side-effects (EPS): muscular rigidity, tremor, slowed motor responses, akathisia (intense restlessness), muscle spasms of head and neck, tardive dyskinesia (TD)
- ✓ Dry mouth
- ✓ Constipation
- ✓ Blurry vision
- ✓ Urinary retention
- ✓ Orthostatic hypotension
- ✓ Weight gain
- ✓ Agranulocytosis
- ✓ Prolactin elevation
- ✓ Elevated triglycerides
- ✓ Type II diabetes
- ✓ Cardiac changes
- ✓ Photosensitivity (sensitivity to sunlight)

Aytpical/Second Generation Antipsychotic Medications

- ✓ Dry mouth
- ✓ Constipation
- ✓ Blurred vision
- ✓ Drowsiness
- ✓ Obesity
- ✓ Diabetes
- ✓ High cholesterol
- ✓ Elevated triglycerides

Schizoaffective Disorder

Schizoaffective disorder combines the symptoms of schizophrenia and the mood symptoms of depression or mania. The symptoms of schizophrenia, however, are noted to occur in the absence of symptoms associated with depression or bipolar for at least two weeks. It is not uncommon, however, for individuals with schizoaffective disorder to be initially misdiagnosed with, particularly, schizophrenia or bipolar disorder.

The treatment of schizoaffective disorder typically includes the use of an antipsychotic medication in combination with a mood stabilizer or an antidepressant. Changing from one antipsychotic to another may help if an individual responds poorly to the first medication or develops intolerable side-effects. The same, of course, is true for the use of mood stabilizers and antidepressants. In addition, psychosocial treatments often serve as a useful adjunct to psychotropic medication. Typically, these involve:

- ✓ Education about the signs and symptoms of schizoaffective disorder.
- ✓ Developing plans of action for when symptoms re-emerge.
- ✓ Developing strategies to cope with symptoms.
- ✓ Developing strategies for improving social skills and/or activities of daily living.

Most individuals with schizoaffective disorder will require life-long treatment with psychotropic medications and psychosocial interventions in order to avoid relapse and maintain optimal functioning. Although limited, research in the form of case studies (Gallucci, Mernaugh, & Dyson, 2004) suggests individuals with intellectual disability and schizoaffective disorder can benefit from the same treatments as those used for individuals without an intellectual disability.

Borderline Personality Disorder

Borderline Personality Disorder (BPD) is a disorder that affects a person's mood, self-image, and relationships. The person's mood may quickly change from joy to sadness or the person may become enraged with little warning. An individual with BPD may feel confused about their identity or direction in life and may have trouble maintaining relationships with others because of their unpredictable behavior.

Prior to concluding a person has BPD, disorders that could cause similar symptoms as those the person is presenting, such as bipolar disorder, generalized anxiety disorder, schizophrenia, or antisocial personality disorder must be ruled-out. It is also important to recognize other disorders the individual may have. For example, many people with BPD also have eating disorders, alcohol or drug problems, anxiety disorder, or depression. These problems can mask BPD and may interfere with treatment if they are not diagnosed and treated.

Symptoms of BPD may vary from person to person, but often include:

- Creating and acting out a crisis to receive attention to avoid feeling abandoned
- Viewing others as all good or all bad
- Frequently changing jobs, friends, and life goals
- Engaging in self destructive behavior like substance abuse, sexual promiscuity, and eating binges
- Attempts to harm themselves through suicide or self-injurious behavior
- Emotional or angry outbursts
- Feelings of unreality or being separated from one's body
- Chronic feelings of emptiness
- Transient psychotic symptoms
- Impulsiveness
- Extreme neediness

Because recognizing the symptoms of borderline personality disorder may be difficult at times, DesNoyers Hurley and Sovner (1988) and Mosley (1999) have offered the following list of behaviors that may be suggestive of the symptoms of BPD in individuals with intellectual disability.

DSM IV-TR SYMPTOMS FOR BPD	PRESENTATION IN SOMEONE WITH INTELLECTUAL DISABILITY
Personal Relationships	• Relationships are volatile • Individual grossly overreacts to staff requests • Use of disturbing slurs against others • Becomes over-attached to a person and then "turns against" them for no obvious reason • Over-idealization of staff or significant others
Impulsivity	• Provoking others • Dangerous sexual activity • Substance abuse • Stealing • Binge eating
Mood Instability	• Extreme change in mood due to minor or nonexistent issue
Poor Anger Control	• Verbal aggression (most frequently) • Physical aggression
Suicidal/Self-Injurious Behavior	• Cutting self with sharp objects • Attempts at suicide

DSM IV-TR SYMPTOMS FOR BPD	PRESENTATION IN SOMEONE WITH INTELLECTUAL DISABILITY
Fear of Abandonment	<ul><li>Repeatedly calling staff/family member on phone (e.g., 10-20 times a day)</li><li>Dramatic acts designed to keep person from leaving</li><li>Unreasonable demands of staff time</li><li>Acts designed to "get rid of" others</li></ul>
Identity Disturbance	<ul><li>Confused or shifting sexual identity</li><li>Stating they are someone other than who they are</li></ul>
Paranoid/Dissociative Symptoms	<ul><li>Statements about others "out to get them"</li><li>Avoidance behaviors</li><li>Bizarre accusations regarding staff</li><li>Non-seizure/neurological periods of confused consciousness</li></ul>

Use of psychotropic medication with individuals with BPD is typically driven by the primary presenting symptoms. For those individuals who primarily experience impulsivity and anger control problems or extreme sensitivity to rejection, SSRIs are frequently prescribed. Mood stabilizers may be used for those individuals with extreme mood lability while low-dose antipsychotics may be used if transient psychosis is noted. In reality, individuals with BPD may need medications from several different classes to assist them in managing the symptoms of their disorder. Treatment also typically includes individual and group therapy, with cognitive and dialectical behavior therapy being the most effective.

Attention Deficit Hyperactivity Disorder

Attention Deficit Hyperactivity Disorder (ADHD) affects approximately five percent of children. Of these children, about two-thirds will continue to experience symptoms into adolescence and adulthood. As these individuals age, there is typically a reduction in restlessness or excessive motor activity. The remaining symptoms of ADHD, however, generally continue into adulthood.

Symptoms of ADHD may vary from person to person, but often include:

- Impulsivity
- Difficulty with motivation
- Distractibility
- Difficulty with concentration and attention
- Difficulty organizing activities
- Restlessness or excessive motor activity
- Difficulty controlling emotions

The primary treatment for ADHD involves the use of stimulants (e.g., methylphenidate, dextroamphetamine). If there is a family history of substance abuse, antidepressants (e.g., buproprion, atomoxetine) or alpha-adrenergic agonists (e.g., clonidine, guanfacine) may be indicated due to the potential for abuse associated with stimulants. Due to the superior efficacy of stimulants, antidepressants and alpha-adrenergic agonists are generally used only in combination with stimulants. It is noted, however, that some individuals will respond favorably to monotherapy with antidepressants or alpha-adrenergic agonists. Moreover, the AAMR Consensus Guidelines (Rush & Frances, 2000) recommend the use of stimulants as the first line of treatment for individuals with ADHD and intellectual disability. Additionally, treatment for ADHD also frequently includes behavior therapy, social skills training, individual and family therapy, and parent or support staff training.

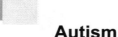

Autism

Individuals with autism will typically have difficulty in four primary areas. These include social interaction, language and communication, adapting to change, and sensory processing. Each of these areas is reviewed in detail below.

Difficulty with Social Interaction

Many individuals with autism do not understand how to interact with others and thus they may tend to avoid being around other people. Difficulties with social interaction range from not being able to tolerate any social contact, to wishing for such contact but not understanding how to handle it.

Behaviors that are suggestive of difficulty with social interaction include:

- Resisting eye contact
- Lacking empathy for others
- Hiding in a corner of a room when others enter
- Avoiding groups
- Standing too close to others
- Not initiating contact with others
- Making socially inappropriate comments
- Moving away when others approach
- Relying on peripheral vision rather than making direct eye contact
- Not understanding jokes or humor
- Using others as functional objects
- Not understanding others' body language or facial expressions

Difficulty with Language

About half of the individuals with autism never speak. Others may be able to speak, but they may not be able to use their language to have a social conversation with others. Often, these individuals will have conversations only about specific areas of interest. Some individuals with autism who speak will be able to use their words to communicate at some times, but not at others. In addition to difficulties with language, many individuals with autism have difficulty understanding the process of communication. In other words, individuals with autism may not understand the process of getting someone's attention, sending a message, waiting for a response, and then responding back.

Behaviors that may be observed that are suggestive of language and communication difficulties include:

- Repeating what others say
- Inconsistent ability to use language
- Inconsistent ability to understand language
- Talking in a sing-song tone of voice
- Not understanding sarcasm, teasing, or idioms
- Being unable to use words

Difficulty with Change

Another characteristic of individuals with autism is that they often experience stress or anxiety when there are changes in their daily routine or environment. Behaviors that may be observed that are suggestive of a difficulty with change include:

- Eating only certain foods
- Wearing certain clothes on certain days
- Wanting activities to occur in a certain order
- Becoming upset with new people (e.g., staff) in environment
- Putting items back in the original place after they have been moved

Difficulty with Sensory Processing

Although people with autism may have normal hearing, vision, smell, and touch, many individuals have difficulty consistently understanding the information coming in from their senses. Behaviors that may be suggestive of sensory processing difficulties include:

- Not sensing pain at times
- Appearing deaf at times
- Covering ears as if sounds are painful
- Becoming overwhelmed in loud environments
- Staring at lights, lines, or spinning objects
- Becoming nauseous due to subtle smells

Use of Medication

Medication is frequently an integral component of treatment for individuals with autism and other pervasive developmental disorders (e.g., Asperger's, PDD-NOS). To be clear, medications are useful only as a means of managing symptoms. Medications do not cure the core deficits noted in autism or the other pervasive developmental disorders. Although not without debate, a variety of medications are used with individuals with autism including:

- ✓ Antipsychotics (risperidone, olanzapine)
- ✓ Antidepressants (anafranil, fluvoxamine)
- ✓ Anti-anxiety medications (buspirone, lorazepam)
- ✓ Mood stabilizers (divalproex)
- ✓ Stimulants (methylphenidate, dextroamphetamine)

With regards to the use of antipsychotic medication, evidence is accumulating in support of the use of atypical antipsychotic medications, particularly risperidone. Well-controlled research has established that the use of risperidone can result in clinically significant reductions in aggression, irritability, repetitive behavior, and anxiety. Although other atypical antipsychotic medications may be used similarly, risperidone is currently the only medication with FDA approval for treatment of the behavioral symptoms associated with autism. Antidepressants, the most widely prescribed psychotropic to individuals with autism, are typically prescribed to treat stereotypies or compulsive behavior. The antidepressants with the most research supporting their use are the SSRIs (e.g., fluvoxamine) and clomipramine. Controlled studies of the stimulants methylphenidate and clonidine suggest these medications may have utility in the treatment of hyperactivity in high-functioning individuals with autism. Potentially significant side-effects (e.g., irritability, hypotension, over-sedation), however, were noted for both of these medications. Other approaches such as the use of anticonvulsant mood stabilizers and anti-anxiety medications may be potentially useful, but definitive research supporting their use is lacking.

Chapter Four

Measuring Efficacy

Psychotropic medications are often initiated without adequate thought as to the specific purpose of the medication, expected outcomes, and the criteria that will be used to evaluate when these outcomes have been achieved. With regard to the question of purpose, it is generally accepted that psychotropic medication should only be prescribed in one of two situations. First, such medication is appropriate when an individual meets the *DSM IV-TR* criteria for a drug-responsive mental health disorder. Second, it is appropriate to prescribe for medication-responsive symptoms or behaviors where the linkage has been established. As an example, chronic over-arousal that contributes to severe challenging behaviors may be addressed through the use of psychotropic medication. It is important to note, however, that the target of the psychotropic medication would be the over-arousal and not the challenging behavior.

Once the purpose of the medication has been identified, it is important to establish systems by which to measure whether the expected outcomes of treatment have been achieved. One way to gauge success is through the use of rating scales developed specifically for individuals with intellectual disability. Ideally, appropriate rating scales would be administered prior to the initiation or adjustment of psychotropic medication and then at regular intervals after the trial or change has begun. Some of the more commonly used rating scales that assess behavior and psychiatric status in individuals with intellectual disability are the following:

Aberrant Behavior Checklist (Aman & Singh, 1986): The ABC is a rating scale that is comprised of 58 items and is divided into five subscales. These subscales include Irritability, Lethargy, Stereotypy, Hyperactivity, and Inappropriate Speech. Although the ABC does not assess for symptomatology consistent with discrete disorders, it is a well-established tool for identifying changes in an individual's behavior secondary to modifications in treatment.

Psychophathology Inventory for Mentally Retarded Adults (Matson, 1997): The PIMRA is a checklist of psychopathological behaviors and is intended for assessment of psychiatric conditions in adolescents and adults with intellectual disability. It is unique in that it includes both an informant rating scale and a self-reporting scale. The PIMRA consists of 56 items divided into eight subscales: Schizophrenia, Affective Disorder, Psychosexual Disorder, Adjustment Disorder, Anxiety Disorder, Somatoform Disorder,

Personality Disorder, and Inappropriate Adjustment. In addition, the PIMRA yields a total score based on all 56 items.

Reiss Screen for Maladaptive Behavior (Reiss, 1988): The *Reiss Screen* is a 38-item scale that screens for mental health problems in persons with an intellectual disability using information supplied by caretakers, teachers, job supervisors, or parents. Totaling 26 of the items provides a score indicating the severity of any psychopathology and thus is well suited as a means of assessing treatment progress. Subscales include Aggressive Behavior, Autism, Psychosis, Paranoia, Depression – Behavioral Signs, Depression – Physical Signs, Dependent Personality Disorder, and Avoidant Personality Disorder. The *Reiss Screen* also includes six maladaptive behavior subscales (drug abuse, overactive, self-injury, sexual problems, stealing, suicidal).

Additional assessment tools that may be of use, as cited in the AAMR's Expert Consensus Guidelines (Rush & Frances, 2000), include:

- ✓ *Conners Parent and Teacher Rating Scales*
- ✓ *Vineland Adaptive Behavior Scale, Part 2*
- ✓ *Child Behavior Checklist*
- ✓ *AAMR Adaptive Behavior Scale, Part 2*
- ✓ *Nisonger Child Behavior Rating Form*
- ✓ *Diagnostic Assessment of the Severely Handicapped*
- ✓ *Reiss Scale for Children's Dual Diagnosis*
- ✓ *Behavioral and Emotional Rating Scale*

Although the widespread use of the above instruments suggests they all have practical or clinical value, there is no consensus as to which is best. Actually, because of the limitations in the scope or psychometric properties of these tools, it is often advisable to complete multiple rating scales. Clinicians responsible for scoring these instruments should use their clinical judgment in assessing the significance of individual test items, as opposed to relying solely on numerical scores.

An alternative, or adjunct, to the use of rating scales is the operational definition of target symptoms, development of data collection systems, and regular summarization of accumulated data. In keeping with this model, King (2006) has described an objective monitoring system for bipolar disorder that combines behavioral equivalents for *DSM IV-TR* diagnostic criteria with specific charting recommendations. The table below provides an example of this type of data collection system.

Bipolar Symptom Monitoring – An Example

DSM IV-TR Symptom	Behavioral Equivalent	Data Collection
Decreased Need for Sleep	Not sleeping, Irregular sleep patterns, Awakens early	Document sleep on data sheet using 15 minute intervals
Irritability	Self-injury, Aggression	Use of Antecedent-Behavior-Consequence (ABC) Tracksheets
Distractibility	Leaves tasks before completion, Can't sit through activities	Track the amount of paychecks from work (paid at piece-rate)

King notes that, optimally, the use of such systems should:

- ✓ Track as many behavioral equivalents as are relevant
- ✓ Include data collection both before and after medication is initiated or changed
- ✓ Track symptoms across all environments
- ✓ Provide for summarization and review of data by the individual and his or her family, as well as the treatment team

Another approach to monitoring for medication efficacy, similar to that described by Pfadt, Korosh, and Wolfson (2003), includes the tracking of symptoms associated with a diagnosed mental health disorder combined with a rating scale that assesses the symptoms' severity. For such a system to be effective, the symptoms tracked must be clearly defined and capable of observation. In addition, the target symptoms must be operationally defined. An example of such a system is shown below.

Bipolar Symptom Monitoring – An Example

DSM IV-TR Symptom	Daily Rating/Date:_____
Irritable (self-injury, aggression)	0 +1 +2 +3
Distractible (leaves tasks before completing, can't sit through activities)	0 +1 +2 +3

0 = Normal/No Problem

+1 = Present but not serious/Minor problem/Infrequent occurrence

+2 = Moderate problem/Required assistance

+3 = Severe problem/Presented a risk to health and safety/Occurred most of the day

As may be apparent, the primary drawback to using this system is the somewhat subjective nature of the ratings. In an effort to ensure the best possible reliability and validity of the data collected in such a system, therefore, the number of raters should be kept to a minimum. In addition, the raters should meet regularly to review scoring criteria and ensure maximum consistency.

In addition to collection of information regarding specific symptomatology, it is also useful to collect data routinely on a person's sleep and appetite. This type of data is important because sleep and appetite disturbances frequently accompany worsening of a person's mental health disorder; these areas also improve upon effective treatment of the disorder.

Usually, the most efficient way to monitor sleep is to complete a "sleep-sheet" in which family members or staff document whether a person is asleep or awake at regular intervals (e.g., every 30 minutes). Appetite can be monitored through the use of food logs, in which everything a person eats is documented, but this approach is so cumbersome that it is seldom implemented consistently. More efficient approaches include collecting data on the percentage of each meal eaten or simple documentation of an individual's weight at regular intervals (e.g., weekly at the same time of day).

Finally, and perhaps most importantly, it is essential that individuals taking psychotropic medication are afforded the opportunity to share their impressions regarding the efficacy of their treatment and their perception of any side-effects. This information, moreover, must be valued and respected. Although the amount of personal data that can be shared may be limited by communication difficulties, this critical indication of effectiveness must never be ignored.

Chapter Five

Monitoring for Side-Effects

Monitoring for medication side-effects is often a difficult task when working with individuals with an intellectual disability. As the severity of intellectual disability increases, such individuals are less likely to be able to report how they feel or how their sense of well-being has changed. Therefore, it is critical that support staff, family members, or a clinician routinely evaluate individuals in a systematic way for the possible presence of physical changes that may be related to the use of medication.

In this regard, a guiding principle in the use of psychotropic medication with individuals with an intellectual disability is that:

The individual must be monitored for side-effects on a regular and systematic basis using an accepted methodology which includes a standardized assessment instrument.

More specifically, this principle means:

- ✓ Standardized assessment tools should be used in addition to any recommended physiological or laboratory assessments
- ✓ Direct examination should accompany use of the assessment instrument
- ✓ Information obtained through standardized assessments should be followed-up on by the evaluating clinician
- ✓ Monitoring should be conducted at least every three to six months, or as clinically appropriate

Multi-system side-effect rating scales that can be used to meet the requirements of the above standard, in part, include the following:

Adverse Drug Reaction Detection Scale (Corso, Pucino, DeLeo, Calis, & Galleil, 1992): The ADRDS is a detailed review of all body parts that is primarily utilized in research or clinical settings.

Dosage Record and Treatment Emergent Symptom Scale (Guy, 1976a): Developed at the National Institute of Mental Health, the DOTES includes a systematic review of all body parts and a physical examination, as well as verbal questions. It too is primarily utilized in research settings.

Subjective Treatment Emergent Symptom Scale (Guy, 1976b): The STESS was designed for use in children up to 15 years of age and can be completed by the parent or care-giver. It can be used to evaluate the presence and severity of an individual's complaints for those who are unable to verbalize them.

Monitoring of Side-effects Scale (Kalachnik, 1988): The MOSES is an assessment for potential medication side-effects that covers 107 different items. It is systematic in that it is structured according to different body systems (e.g., GI, urinary, bowel, sight, hearing), and it may be easily completed by trained care-givers or family members. It is both qualitative (i.e., assessing whether a system is affected) and quantitative (i.e., rating the significance of a problem on scale of 1 to 5). This scale should be completed at baseline (for later comparison) and at least every three months thereafter or more frequently if medications are being adjusted or changed. Portions of the MOSES also allow for narrative statements if needed for clarification.

Other side-effect specific rating scales include the following:

Assessment of Involuntary Movement Scale (Guy, 1976c): Developed by the National Institute of Mental Health, the AIMS is a 12-item instrument to assess and quantify abnormal movements in different parts of the body in adults, children, and adolescents.

Akathisia Rating Movement Scale (Bodfish, Newell, Sprage, Harper, & Lewis, 1997): The ARMS is utilized to assess akathisia or restlessness in persons with developmental disabilities.

Dyskinesia Identification System – Condensed User Scale (Sprague & Kalachnik, 1991): The DISCUS is a tool to measure and quantify tardive dyskinesia, and is uniquely tailored to assess abnormal movements in persons with developmental disabilities. This assessment instrument has been validated in persons with developmental disabilities. Scores are highly correlated with the presence of tardive dyskinesia. The DISCUS, however, does not capture symptoms of tardive akathesia.

Barnes Akathesia Rating Scale (Barnes, 1989): Trained clinicians utilize the BARS to evaluate and quantify the presence of drug-induced akathesia or restlessness in adults, children, and adolescents.

Simpson Angus Scale (Simpson & Angus, 1970): The SAS is utilized to measure and quantify drug-induced Parkinsonism or extrapyramidal effects in adults, children, and adolescents, such as rigidity, tremor, and salivation.

Consistent collection of information using the above instruments can play a vital role in the evaluation of the individual's overall physical quality of life, as well as assessing the evolution of potential medication side-effects. Unwanted effects associated with possible classes of medication that individuals, families, and support staff should watch for include but may not be limited to the following:

Selective Serotonin Reuptake Inhibitors (SSRI)

- ✓ Difficulty sleeping
- ✓ Increase in anxiousness or restlessness
- ✓ Nausea
- ✓ Diarrhea
- ✓ Headaches
- ✓ Reduced sexual interest or sexual dysfunction
- ✓ Potentially dangerous reaction when combine with MAOIs

Tricylic (TCA) Antidepressants

- ✓ Dry mouth
- ✓ Constipation
- ✓ Difficulty urinating
- ✓ Light headedness
- ✓ Blurred vision
- ✓ Urinary retention
- ✓ Dizziness

Monamine Oxidase Inhibitors (MAOI) Antidepressants

- ✓ Weight gain
- ✓ Dizziness
- ✓ Reduced sexual interest or sexual dysfunction
- ✓ Potentially deadly hypertensive reaction when combined with certain foods or medications containing tyrosine (e.g., aged cheese, red wine, coffee, cold remedies, chocolate)

Serotonin and Norepinephrine Reuptake Inhibitor Antidepressants (SNRI)

- ✓ Nausea
- ✓ Sexual dysfunction
- ✓ Sweating
- ✓ Sleep disturbance
- ✓ Increased blood pressure

Lithium

- ✓ Nausea
- ✓ Diarrhea
- ✓ Vomiting
- ✓ Hand tremor
- ✓ Polyuria (excessive urination)
- ✓ Polydispsia (excessive thirst)
- ✓ Edema
- ✓ Dry mouth
- ✓ Cardiac conduction abnormality

Side-effects of chronic, or long term, lithium use include:

- ✓ Hypothyroidism
- ✓ Kidney damage

Signs of lithium toxicity include:

- ✓ Lethargy
- ✓ Slurred speech
- ✓ Ringing in the ears
- ✓ Vomiting
- ✓ Tremor
- ✓ Seizures
- ✓ Delirium
- ✓ Ataxia

Anticonvulsant Mood Stabilizers

- ✓ Nausea
- ✓ Sedation
- ✓ Weight gain
- ✓ Rashes
- ✓ Hand tremor
- ✓ Blood dyscrasias
- ✓ Ataxia

Atypical Antipsychotics:

- ✓ Dry mouth
- ✓ Constipation
- ✓ Blurred vision
- ✓ Drowsiness
- ✓ Weight gain
- ✓ Type II diabetes
- ✓ Elevated Triglycerides
- ✓ Agranulocytosis
- ✓ Extrapyramidal Side-effects (EPS): muscular rigidity, tremor, slowed motor responses, akathisia (intense restlessness), muscle spasms of head and neck, tardive dyskinesia (TD)
- ✓ Cardiac QTC prolongation

Typical Antipscyhotics:

- ✓ Extrapyramidal Side-effects (EPS): muscular rigidity, tremor, slowed motor responses, akathisia (intense restlessness), muscle spasms of head and neck, tardive dyskinesia (TD)
- ✓ Dry mouth
- ✓ Constipation
- ✓ Blurry vision
- ✓ Urinary retention
- ✓ Weight gain
- ✓ Cardiac conduction abnormalities
- ✓ Photosensitivity (sensitivity to sunlight)

ADHD Therapies

- ✓ Reduced appetite, weight loss
- ✓ Nausea and vomiting
- ✓ Headache
- ✓ Irritability or jitteriness
- ✓ Rebound symptoms

This long list of possible drug reactions does not mean that psychotropic medication is too dangerous to be given to persons with intellectual disabilities. Rather, it means that vigilance in monitoring for the possible emergence of negative side-effects is extremely important.

Psychotropic Medications – A Partial Listing

ANTIDEPRESSANTS/ANTIOBSESSIONALS

Trade Name	Generic Name	Category
Celexa	Citalopram	SSRI
Cymbalta	Duloxetine	SNRI
Desyrel	Trazodone	Other
Effexor	Venlafaxine	SNRI
Elavil	Amitriptyline	TCA
Emsam	Selegiline transdermal	MAOI
Lexapro	Escitalopram	SSRI
Luvox	Fluvoxamine	SSRI
Pamelor	Nortriptyline	TCA
Parnate	Tranylcypromine	MAOI
Paxil	Paroxetine	SSRI
Prozac	Fluoxetine	SSRI
Remeron	Mirtazapine	Other
Serzone	Nefazodone	Other
Sinequan	Doxepin	TCA
Tofranil	Imipramine	TCA
Wellbutrin	Bupropion	Other
Zoloft	Sertraline	SSRI

ANTIPSYCHOTICS

Atypical/Second Generation

Trade Name	Generic Name
Abilify	Aripiprazole
Clozaril	Clozapine
Geodon	Ziprasidone
Invega	Paliperidone
Risperdal	Risperidone
Seroquel	Quetiapine
Symbyax	Olanzapine/Fluoxetine
Zyprexa	Olanzapine

Typical/First Generation

Trade Name	Generic Name
Haldol	Haloperidol
Loxitane	Loxapine

Trade Name	Generic Name
Mellaril	Thioridazine
Moban	Molindone
Navane	Thiothixene
Orap	Pimozide
Prolixin	Fluphenazine
Serentil	Mesoridazine
Stelazine	Trifluoperazine
Thorazine	Chlorpromazine
Trilafon	Perphenazine

MOOD STABILIZERS

Trade Name	Generic Name
Depakene	Valproic Acid
Depakote	Divalproex
Eskalith	Lithium
Lamictal	Lamotrigine
Neurontin	Gabapentin
Tegretol	Carbamazepine
Topamax	Topiramate
Trileptal	Oxcarbazepine

ANTIANXIETY

Trade Name	Generic Name
Ativan	Lorazepam
Buspar	Buspirone
Klonopin	Clonazepam
Librium	Chlordiazepoxide
Serax	Oxazepam
Tranxene	Clorazepate
Valium	Diazepam
Vistaril	Hydroxyzine
Xanax	Alprazolam

HYPNOTICS

Trade Name	Generic Name
Ambien	Zolpidem
Benadryl	Diphenhydramine
Dalmane	Flurazepam
Halcion	Triazolam
Lunesta	Eszopiclone

Trade Name	Generic Name
Noctec	Chloral Hydrate
Restoril	Temazepam
Rozerem	Ramelteon
Sonata	Zaleplon

ANTIPARKINSONIAN

Trade Name	Generic Name
Artane	Trihexyphenidyl
Cogentin	Benztropine
Symmetrel	Amantadine

ADHD THERAPIES

Trade Name	Generic Name
Dexedrine	Dextroamphetamine
Ritalin, Concerta	Methylphenidate
Strattera	Atomoxetine
Adderal	Mixed amphetamine/dextroamphetamine salts

References

Altabet, S., Neumann, K., & Watson-Johnson. (2002). Light therapy as a treatment of sleep cycle problems and depression. *Mental Health Aspects of Developmental Disabilities*, 5-1, 1-6.

Aman, M.G., & Singh, N.N. (1986). *Aberrant Behavior Checklist*. East Aurora, NY: Slosson Educational Publications, Inc.

American Psychiatric Association (2000). *Diagnostic and statistical manual of mental disorders, Fourth edition, Text Revision*. Washington, DC: Author.

Barnes, T.R. (1989). A rating scale for drug-induced akathisia. *British Journal of Psychiatry*, 154, 672-676.

Bates, W.J., Smeltzer, D.J., & Arnockzy, S. (1986). Appropriate and Inappropriate use of psychotherapeutic medications for institutionalized mentally retarded persons. *American Journal of Mental Deficiency*, 90, 363-370.

Bodfish, J.W, & Madison, J.T. (1993). Diagnosis and fluoxetine treatment of Compulsive behavior disorder of adults with mental retardation. *American Journal on Mental Retardation*. 98, 360-367.

Bodfish, J.W., Newell KM, Sprague RL, Harper, V.N., & Lewis, M.H. (1997). Akathisia in Adults with Mental Retardation: Development of the Akathisia Ratings of Movement Scale (ARMS). *American Journal of Mental Retardation,* 101: 413-423.

Boulding, R., Friedlander R., Jurenka, S., Hrynchak, M., & Honer, W. (2005). Early onset schizophrenia in a young woman with mild intellectual disability and unbalanced chromosomal translocation. *Mental Health Aspects of Developmental Disabilities*, 8-2, 40-44.

Burgess, L.H., (2002). Gabapentin: An alternative mood stabilizer for patients with developmental disabilities. *Mental Health Aspects of Developmental Disabilities,* 5-1, 22-24.

Charlot, L.R. (1997). Developmental effects on psychiatric disorders in persons with mental retardation. In McNelis, D.N. & McNelis, T.M. (Eds.) *Conference Proceedings, 14th Annual NADD Conference*. Kingston, NY: NADD.

Cook, E.H., Terry, E.J., Heller, W., & Leventhal, B.L. (1990). Fluoxetine treatment of borderline mentally retarded adults with obsessive-compulsive disorder. *Journal of Clinical Psychopharmacology*, 10, 228-229.

Corso, D.M., Pucino, F., DeLeo, J.M., Calis, K.A., & Galleil, J.F. (1992). Development of a questionairre for detecting potential adverse drug reactions. *Annals of Pharmacotherapy. 26*, 890-896.

DesNoyers Hurley, A. & Sovner, R. (1988). The clinical characteristics and management of borderline personality disorder in mentally retarded persons. *Psychiatric Aspects of Mental Retardation Reviews*, 7-7&8.

Dimascio, A. (1975). Psychotropic drug usage in the mentally retarded: A review of 2000 cases. In Reiss & Aman (Eds.), *The international consensus handbook*, 31. USA: Ohio State University Nisonger Center.

Findholt, N.E., & Emmett, C.G. (1990). Impact of interdisciplinary team review on psychotropic drug use with persons who have mental retardation. *Mental Retardation*, 28, 41-46.

Fletcher, R.J., & Dosen, A. (1993). *Mental health aspects of mental retardation.* New York: Lexington Books.

Gedye, A. (1992). Recognizing obsessive-compulsive disorders in clients with developmental disabilities. *The Habilitative Mental Healhcare Newsletter*, 11-11.

Gallucci, G., Mernaugh, L., & Dyson, D. (2004). Ariprrazole use an individual with intellectual disability and schizoaffective disorder. *Mental Health Aspects of Developmental Disabilities*, 7-2, 53-56.

Gualtieri, C. T. (1988). Mental health aspects of persons with mental retardation. In J.A. Stark, F.J. Menolascino, M.H. Albarelli, & Y.C. Gray (Eds.), *Mental retardation and mental health.* New York: Springer-Verlag.

Guy W. (1976a). Dosage Record and Treatment Emergent Symptom Scale. In *ECDEU assessment manual for psychopharmacology.* Rev. (DHEW Publication Number ADM 76-338, pp. 223-44). Rockville, MD: U.S. National Institute of Health, Psychopharmacology Research Branch.

Guy W. (1976b). Subjective Treatment Emergent Symptom scale. In *ECDEU Assessment Manual for Psychopharmacology* (revised). Department of Health, Education, and Human Welfare Publication No. (ADM) 76-338, pp. 347-350. Rockville, MD.

Guy W. (1976c). Abnormal Involuntary Movement Scale. In *ECDEU Assessment Manual for Psychopharmacology*, revised (DHEW publication number ADM-76-338, pp 534-37). Washington, DC, US Department of Health, Education, and Welfare.

Heistad, G.T., Simmerman, R.L., & Doebler, M.J. (1982). Long-term usefulness of thioridazine for institutionalized mentally retarded patients. *American Journal of Mental Deficiency*, 87, 243-251.

Hurley, A. (1999). Psychotic features in persons with mental retardation. In Fletcher, R.J., Griffiths, D., & Nagy-McNelis, D. (Eds.), *Proceedings, 16th annual NADD conference*. Kingston, NY: NADD.

Hurley, A.D., Folstein, M., & Lam, N. (2003). Patients with and without intellectual disabilities seeking outpatient psychiatric services: Diagnoses and prescribing patterns. *Journal of Intellectual Disability Research*, 47, 39-50.

Kalachnik, J.E. (1988). *Medication monitoring procedures: thou shall, here's how*, in Gadow K.D , Poling, A. G., Eds. *Pharmacotherapy and Mental Retardation*, College-Hill: Boston, MA. p. 231-268.

King, R. (2006). Charting for a purpose – phase II: Optimal treatment of bipolar disorder in individuals with developmental disabilities. *Mental Health Aspects of Developmental Disabilities*, 9-2, 54-68.

Laman, D.S., & Reiss, S. (1987). Social skill deficiencies associated with depressed mood of mentally retarded adults. *American Journal of Mental Deficiency*, 92, 224-229.

LaMendola, R.S., Zaharia, E.S., & Carver, M. (1980). Reducing psychotropic drug use in an institution for the retarded. *Hospital and Community Psychiatry*, 31, 243-245.

Lew, M. (1995). Behavioral approaches to working with obsessive-compulsive disorder in persons with mental retardation. *The Habilitative Mental Healthcare Newsletter. 14-5*.

Lipman, R.S. (1970). The use of psychopharmacological agents in residential facilities for the retarded. In F.J. Menolascino (Ed.), *Psychiatric approaches to mental retardation*, 382-389. New York: Basic Books.

Lowry, M.A. (1995). Anger: A root of problem behavior in the depressed. *The Habilitative Mental Healthcare Newsletter. 14-6*.

Lowry, M.A. (1997) Unmasking mood disorders: Recognizing and measuring symptomatic behaviors. *The Habilitative Mental Healthcare Newsletter.16-1*.

Matson, J.L. (1988). *The Psychopathology Inventory for Mentally Retarded Adults*. Worthington, OH: IDS Publishing Corp.

Matson, J.L. (1995). *The diagnostic assessment for the severely handicapped – revised (DASH-II).* Baton Rouge, LA: Scientific Publishers.

Matson, J.L. (1997). *The assessment of dual diagnosis (ADD).* Baton Rouge, LA: Scientific Publishers.

Mavromatis, M.I. (1999). Two case reports of premenstrual dysphoric disorder in women with mental retardation. *Mental Health Aspects of Developmental Disabilities*, 2-3, 92-94.

McGuire, D.E. & Chicoine, B.A. (1996). Depressive disorders in adults with down syndrome. *The Habilitative Healthcare Newsletter, 1, 1-7.*

Mosley, K. (1999). Underdiagnosed, but ever present: Borderline personality in persons with developmental disabilities. In Fletcher, R.J., Griffiths, D., & Nagy-McNelis, D. (Eds.) *Proceedings – 16th annual NADD conference.*

Myers, B.A. & Peuschel, S.M. (1993). Differentiating schizophrenia from other mental disorders and behavioral disorders in persons with developmental disabilties. *The Habilitative Mental Healthcare Newsletter*, 12-6.

Nezu, C.M., Nezu, A.M., & Gill-Wiess, M.J. (1992). *Psychopathology in persons with mental retardation: Clinical guidelines for assessment and treatment.* Champaign, IL: Research Press.

Pary, R., Friedlander, R., & Capone G. (1999). Bipolar disorder and down syndrome: Six cases. *Mental Health Aspects of Developmental Disabilities*, 2-2, 59-63.

Pfadt, A., Korosh, W., & Wolfson, M. (2003). Charting bipolar disorder in people With developmental disabilities: An informant based tracking system. *Mental Health Aspects of Developmental Disabilities*, 6-1, 1-10.

Reiss, S. (1994). *Handbook of challenging behavior: Mental health aspects of mental retardation.* Worthington, OH: IDS Publishing.

Reiss, S. (1988). *The Reiss Screen for Maladaptive Behavior.* Worthington, OH: IDS Publishing Corp.

Reiss, S. & Aman, M. (1998). *Psychotropic medication and developmental disabilties:* The international consensus handbook. Columbus, OH: The Ohio State University Nisonger Clinic.

Reiss, S. & Rojahn. (1993). Joint occurrence of depression and aggression in children and adults with mental retardation. *Journal of Intellectual Disabilities*, 37, 1116-1125.

Reiss, S., Levitan, G.W., & Szysko, J. (1982). Emotional disturbance and mental retardation: Diagnostic overshadowing. *American Journal of Mental Deficiency, 86*, 396-402.

Rush, A.J. & Frances, A. (Eds.) (2000). Expert consensus guideline series: Treatment of psychiatric and behavioral problems in mental retardation. *American Journal on Mental Retardation*, 105 (3).

Ryan, R.M. (1996). *Handbook of mental health care for persons with developmental disabilities*. Evergreen, CO: S&B Publishing.

Shalock, R.L., Foley, J.W., Toulouse, A., & Stark, J.A. (1985). Medication and programming in controlling the behavior of mentally retarded individuals in community settings. *American Journal of Mental Deficiency*, 89, 503-509.

Simpson, G.M. and J.W. Angus. (1970). A rating scale for extrapyramidal side effects. *Acta Psychiatrica Scandinavica Supplement*, 212, 11-19.

Sobsey, D. & Varnhagen, C. (1991). Sexual abuse and exploitation of Canadians with disabilities. In Bagley, C. & Thomlinson, R.J. (Eds.) *Child sexual abuse: Critical perspectives on prevention, intervention, and treatment.* Toronto: Wall and Emerson.

Sovner, R. & Lowrey, M.A. (1990). A behavioral methodology for diagnosing affective disorders in indviduals with mental retardation. *The Habilitative Mental Healthcare Newsletter*, 9-7.

Sovner, R., Foz, C.J., Lowry, M.J., & Lowry, M.A. (1993). Fluoxetine treatment of depression and associated self-injury in two adults with mental retardation. *Journal of Intellectual Disability Research*, 37, 301-311.

Sprague, R.I. Kalachnik, J.E. (1991). Reliability and a total score cutoff for the Dyskinesia Identification System: Condensed User Scale (DISCUS) with mentally ill and mentally retarded populations. *Psychopharmacology Bulletin*, 27, 51-58.

Spreat, S., Conroy, J.W., & Fullerton, A. (2004). Statewide longitudinal survey of psychotropic medication use for persons with mental retardation. *American Journal on Mental Retardation*, 109-4, 322-331.

Suppes, T. & Dennehy, E.B. (2005). *Bipolar disorder: The latest assessment and treatment strategies*. Kansas City, MO: Dean Psych Press Corp.

Tu, J.B. & Smith, J.T. (1979). A survey of psychotropic medication in mental retardation facilities. *Journal of Clinical Psychiatry,* 40, 125-128.

Vitiello, B., Spreat, S., & Behar, D. (1989). Obsessive-compulsive disorder in mentally retarded patients. *Journal of Nervous and Mental Disease*, 177, 232-236.

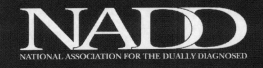

NATIONAL ASSOCIATION FOR THE DUALLY DIAGNOSED

132 Fair St., Kingston, NY 12401-4802
Phone (845) 331-4336 • (800) 331-5362
Fax (845) 331-4569
e-mail: info@thenadd.org
www.thenadd.org

Join NADD today!

It's easy to sign up:
Just go to **www.thenadd.org**

Membership Matters and You Make a Difference!

Members are an integral part of what makes the National Association for the Dually Diagnosed (NADD) a leader in the dissemination of state-of-the-art information. When joining NADD you will immediately be recognized as an individual who is concerned about the issues facing mental health care for persons who have intellectual disabilities. Simply by joining NADD you will become a prestigious member and have a voice in NADD's growing influential organization.

We invite you to join NADD today and build knowledge.

NADD is the leading organization providing professionals, educators, policy makers and families with education, training and information on mental health issues relating to persons with intellectual disabilities.

Education is important and NADD provides members with opportunity to learn more:

- Regional Conferences
- Annual Conferences
- International Conferences
- Teleconference Training
- Online Training (Continuing Education Credits)
- Onsite Consulting/Training for Government/Private Organizations

NADD Members receive discounts on all services and products

Over >>

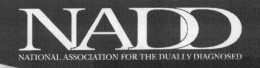
NATIONAL ASSOCIATION FOR THE DUALLY DIAGNOSED

www.thenadd.org

Added Value to Your Membership

■ **Free Subscription** to *The NADD Bulletin*
Included in your membership is a subscription to *The NADD Bulletin*. Each of the six issues per year contains best practice articles by experts in the field. This publication is one of the best known resources for disseminating information on relevent issues.

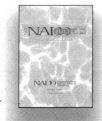

■ **Free subscription** to the *Journal of Mental Health Research in Intellectual Disabilities* (begins 2008)
The *Journal of Mental Health Research in Intellectual Disabilities*, the official research journal of NADD, is soliciting articles in a variety of fields. The journal will accept a wide range of scholarly contributions with an emphasis on empirically-based research.

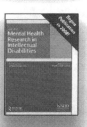

Training & Educational Products
NADD publishes the world's largest selection of training products on persons with intellectual disabilities and mental health needs including books, DVDs, CDs, videos and audiotapes.

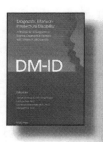
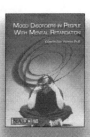
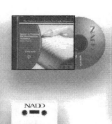
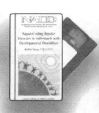
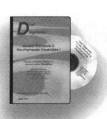

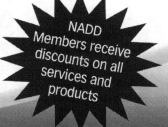
NADD Members receive discounts on all services and products